Surgery in Breast Cancer and Melanoma

Handbooks in General Surgery

D0851230

Kirby I. Bland • Michael G. Sarr
Markus W. Büchler • Attila Csendes
O. James Garden • John Wong
Editors

Surgery in Breast Cancer and Melanoma

Handbooks in General Surgery

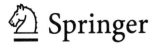 Springer

Editors

Kirby I. Bland, MD
Fay Fletcher Kerner Professor
and Chairman
Department of Surgery
Deputy Director
Comprehensive Cancer Center
University of Alabama School
of Medicine
Birmingham, AL, USA

Markus W. Büchler, MD
Professor of Surgery
and Chairman
Department of General
and Visceral Surgery
University of Heidelberg
Heidelberg, Germany

Attila Csendes, MD, FACS (Hon)
Professor of Surgery
and Chairman
Department of Surgery
University Hospital
Santiago, Chile

Michael G. Sarr, MD
James C. Mason Professor
of Surgery
Department of Surgery
Mayo Clinic College of
Medicine
Rochester, MN, USA

O. James Garden, MBChB, MD,
FRCS (Ed), FRCP (Ed),
FRACS (Hon)
Regius Professor of Clinical
Surgery
Department of Clinical and
Surgical Sciences
The University of Edinburgh
Royal Infirmary of Edinburgh
Edinburgh, UK

John Wong, BSc (Med (Syd)),
MBBS (Syd),
PhD (Syd), MD (Hon (Syd)),
FRACS, FRCS (Edin),
FRCS (Glasg),
FACS (Hon)
Chair Professor
Department of Surgery
The University of Hong Kong
Queen Mary Hospital
Hong Kong, China

ISBN 978-1-84996-434-0   e-ISBN 978-1-84996-435-7

DOI 10.1007/978-1-84996-435-7

Springer London Dordrecht Heidelberg New York

British Library Cataloguing in Publication Data

A catalogue record for this book is available from the British Library

Library of Congress Control Number: 2010938114

Springer is part of Springer Science+Business Media (www.springer.com)

Preface

The editors designed the original textbook *General Surgery: Principles and International Practice* from which this shorter paperback monograph on oncological surgery was taken to be an accessible, concise, and state-of-the-art volume that explores and documents evolutionary principles in the practice of surgery. This work is aimed at the general surgeon and the resident in training. The scientific community continues to witness extraordinary advances in the therapy of both benign and malignant surgical diseases of various organ sites. Much of this progress has been evident over the past decade with new concepts and techniques of management that allow the surgeon to integrate this discipline with medicine, pharmacology, immunology, biostatistics, pathology, genetics, medical and radiation oncology, and diagnostic radiology and imaging. Further, each of these major disciplines contributes a small component for the diagnostic and therapeutic approaches to clinical care; hence the comprehensive planning, integration, and provision of patient care throughout the preoperative, intraoperative, and postoperative phases of care remains essential in the successful practice of our specialty.

The editors acknowledge that the aim of this work is to provide an illustrative, instructive, and comprehensive review that depicts the rationale of basic operative principles essential to surgical therapy. In organizing this monograph, the editors chose authors renowned in the disciplines for illustrating, forming, and depicting in a comprehensive fashion the surgical therapy expectant for metabolic, infectious, endocrine, and neoplastic abnormalities in adult and pediatric patients **from a truly international and multi-continental perspective.** The editors and authors were chosen carefully from across geographies and also from multi-cultural and diverse locations. While the authors consider this text to be inclusive regarding the technical and operative conditions for perioperative care in this field, its purpose should not be intended to replace standard textbooks of surgery nor should it be considered complete in its coverage of pathophysiologic disorders. In contrast, this monograph is organized to familiarize practicing surgeons, residents, and fellows with state-of-the-art surgical principles and techniques essential to contemporary practice. Therefore, the tenor of this monograph on oncological surgery has been developed to coexist with other major surgical reference texts that are dedicated—some in more comprehensive fashion—to the therapy of individual organs of systemic diseases. This monograph is much more a "working text" for the practicing surgeon with emphasis on diagnosis and treatment of oncological disorders. Along with this monograph, nine other paperback monographs are available and focus on the general principles of surgery, trauma, critical care, esophagus and stomach, small bowel, colorectal, liver and biliary, pancreas and spleen, and endocrine organs, all adapted from the primary textbook— *General Surgery: International Principles and Practice.*

The chapters in this monograph on oncological surgery include a condensed bibliography of highly selective journal articles, reviews, and text. In this manner of attempting to be concise, we hope to provide a precise focus for the education of the reader relative to accepted surgical principles involved in patient care. Moreover, the editors have sought to provide a counterpoint view for the selection of therapy by presenting at the opening of each chapter a list of "Pearls and Pitfalls" that highlight particular concerns or controversies. The chapters provide pertinent, though not exhaustive, summaries of anatomy and physiology, a history of surgical illness, and stages of operative approaches with relevant technical considerations outlined in an easily understandable manner. Complications are reviewed when appropriate for the organ system, diseases, and problem. The text is supported amply by line drawings and photographs that depict anatomic or technical principles. The editors have made every attempt to minimize duplicative or repetitive discussions except when controversial or state-of-the-art issues are presented. Moreover, the editors have attempted to ensure that accurate presentations and illustrations depict properly the most complex problems confronted by the general surgeon.

Finally, in an attempt to address advances in contemporary concepts, the text has been organized to address in detail expeditious, safe, and anatomically accurate operations and incorporate standard as well as evolving surgical principles and techniques. These principles have been tested in the clinics of valid scientific knowledge and are well supported by the time-tested approaches that have been provided by practicing surgeons. The editors are excited to be able to respond to the challenge of developing a truly international text and are indeed hopeful that our readers will find this focused monograph on oncological surgery to be a repository of insight, useful, and timely information.

Kirby I. Bland
Michael G. Sarr
Markus W. Büchler
Attila Csendes
O. James Garden
John Wong

Contents

Contributors

Patricio Andrades, MD
Research Associate, Department of Surgery, University
of Alabama at Birmingham, Birmingham, AL, USA

Nimmi Arora, MD
Research Fellow, Division of General Surgery,
Department of Surgery, New York Presbyterian Hospital,
New York, NY, USA

Charles M. Balch, MD, FACS
Professor of Surgery, Oncology & Dermatology, Deputy
Director for Clinical Trials & Outcomes, Johns Hopkins
Institute for Clinical & Translational Research, Johns
Hopkins Medicine, Baltimore, MD, USA

Glen C. Balch, MD
Assistant Professor, Department of Surgery, Memorial Sloan
Kettering Cancer Center, New York, NY, USA

Kirby I. Bland, MD
Fay Fletcher Kerner Professor and Chairman, Department
of Surgery Deputy Director, Comprehensive Cancer Center,
University of Alabama School of Medicine, Birmingham,
AL, USA

Susan W. Caro, MSN, RNC, APNG
Director, Family Cancer Risk Service, Vanderbilt-Ingram Cancer Center, Vanderbilt University Medical Center, Nashville, TN, USA

Steven L. Chen, MD, MBA
Department of Surgical Oncology, John Wayne Cancer Institute, Santa Monica, CA, USA

Eugene A. Choi, MD
Instructor in General Surgery, Department of Surgical Oncology, University of Texas, Houston, TX, USA

J. Michael Dixon, BSc(Hon), MBChB, MD, FRCSEng, FRCSEd, FRCPEd(Hon)
Consultant Surgeon and Senior Lecturer in Surgery, Edinburgh Breast Unit, Western General Hospital, Edinburgh, UK

Mark B. Faries, MD
Director, Translational Tumor Immunology, Department of Surgical Oncology, John Wayne Cancer Institute, Santa Monica, CA, USA

Theresa A. Graves, MD
Assistant Professor, Department of Surgery, Brown University Medical School, Providence, RI, USA

Jhanelle Gray, MD
Assistant Professor, Department of Medical Oncology, H. Lee Moffitt Cancer Center and Research Institute, Tampa, FL, USA

Ajay Jain, MD
Assistant Professor, Department of Surgery, Johns Hopkins University, Baltimore, MD, USA

V. Suzanne Klimberg, MD
Professor, Department of Surgery, Chief, Breast Surgical
Oncology, University of Arkansas for Medical Sciences,
Little Rock, AR, USA

Aleksandra Kuciejewska, MRCP
Breast Unit, Royal Marsden London, London, UK

Julie R. Lange, MD, ScM
Assistant Professor of Surgery and Oncology, Department
of Surgery, Johns Hopkins Medicine, Baltimore, MD, USA

Stanley P. L. Leong, MD, FACS
Professor, Department of Surgery, University of California,
San Francisco, CA, USA

Kelly M. McMasters, MD, PhD
Sam and Lolita Weakley Professor and Chairman,
Department of Surgery, University of Louisville School of
Medicine, Louisville, KY, USA

Donald L. Morton, MD
Chief, Melanoma Program, John Wayne Cancer Institute,
Santa Monica, CA, USA

Emma L. Murray, MBChB, BSc Hons
Edinburgh Breast Unit, Western General Hospital,
Edinburgh, UK

Pamela N. Munster, MD
Medical Oncologist, Department of Interdisciplinary
Oncology, H. Lee Moffitt Cancer Center and Research
Institute, Tampa, FL, USA

David L. Page, MD
Professor of Pathology and Preventive Medicine,
Department of Pathology, Vanderbilt University Medical
Center, Nashville, TN, USA

Raphael E. Pollock, MD, PhD
Division Head, Surgery Department of Surgical Oncology,
University of Texas M D Anderson Center, Houston, TX,
USA

Laurence Z. Rosenberg, MD, BS
Southeastern Plastic Surgery and Department of Surgery,
Florida State University School of Medicine, Tallahassee,
FL, USA

Rache M. Simmons, MD, FACS
Associate Professor, Department of Surgery, New York
Presbyterian Hospital, Weill Medical College, New York,
NY, USA

Ian E. Smith, MD, FRCP, FRCPE
Professor of Cancer Medicine, Royal Marsden Hospital
London, London, UK

Margaret Thompson, MD
Breast Fellow and Instructor, Department of Surgery/
Division of Breast Surgical, University of Arkansas for
Medical Sciences Little Rock, AR, USA

Marshall M. Urist, MD
Professor of Surgical Oncology, Department of Surgery,
University of Alabama at Birmingham, Birmingham, AL,
USA

Luis O. Vasconez, MD
Professor and Director, Division of Plastic Surgery,
Department of Surgery, University of Alabama at
Birmingham, Birmingham, AL, USA

Part I
Breast

1
Benign Breast Disease: Diagnosis and Assessment

Margaret Thompson and V. Suzanne Klimberg

Pearls and Pitfalls

- One of the most important aspects of evaluating a benign breast mass is to rule out a malignancy.
- Never assume a younger woman's breast complaint is benign.
- The best treatment for mastalgia is to alleviate the concern for breast cancer.
- A thorough physical examination should include the entire breast, chest wall, back, and the lymph nodes (axilla, supraclavicular, infraclavicular, and cervical).
- When evaluating breast pain, be sure to do a comprehensive history and physical to exclude bursitis, musculoskeletal disorders, and referred pain from the abdomen.
- A breast mass with any suspicious characteristics should be biopsied even if imaging studies are normal. Always obtain tissue (via biopsy) with concern of malignancy.
- The most important aspect of managing mastitis is follow-up, to ensure it has resolved and is not inflammatory breast cancer.
- Ultrasound remains a very valuable diagnostic tool to the breast surgeon, in the clinic, at the bedside, and in the operating room.
- Despite the development of new biopsy devices and techniques, choose the one that is most appropriate for the particular biopsy you are performing and your particular

K.I. Bland et al. (eds.), *Surgery in Breast Cancer and Melanoma*, DOI 10.1007/978-1-84996-435-7_1, © Springer-Verlag London Limited 2011

practice needs. You may need more than one type of biopsy device to cover all situations.

• Masses with triple-negative results (benign physical exam, imaging studies, and biopsy) should be observed.

Summary

Most breast problems are benign, and include a wide array of discrete pathologies. Although benign, they can also be associated with discomfort, anxiety about cancer, and affect cosmesis; therefore, they require thorough work-up and treatment.

The most common benign breast condition is called fibrocystic changes (FCC). This is commonly called fibrocystic disease because it is so prevalent and is considered part of the natural history of the breast; it is truly not a disease. FCC are nodular fibroglandular tissue and typically present as mastalgia and breast tenderness. FCC is most commonly seen in women ages 35–45, in contrast to fibroadenomas that are typically seen in younger women ages 15–25. Fibroadenomas are usually well circumscribed, non-tender, firm, and mobile.

Mastalgia, or breast pain, is arguably the most common reason women seek medical attention. The cause is unknown, but both benign and malignant diseases can present as breast pain, and thus pain warrants evaluation. Cardiac, abdominal, and musculoskeletal sources should also be investigated, as they can cause referred pain to the breast.

Benign ductal conditions, duct ectasia or intraductal papillomas, may present in a similar fashion. Both can have clear, bloody, or non-bloody discharge. In addition, duct ectasia can present as an infection if the lining of the duct becomes ulcerated. Mastitis and abscesses can present similarly, with warmth, tenderness, and redness. Follow-up of these benign conditions is mandatory to avoid missing a diagnosis of inflammatory breast cancer.

Some benign breast conditions have a higher risk for the development of malignancy. Atypical hyperplasia can increase a women's risk of breast cancer by more than fourfold, and as much as ninefold, if associated with a family history of breast cancer. Atypical hyperplasia can sometimes be difficult to distinguish from lobular carcinoma in situ (LCIS) and ductal carcinoma in situ (DCIS). Papillomas have shown an increased risk of cancer, especially if associated with atypical hyperplasia. Women with papilloma and atypical hyperplasia have a higher risk of developing a subsequent DCIS than those papillomas without atypia. This chapter will discuss the diagnosis and assessment of benign breast disease.

Patient History

One of the most important aspects of evaluating a benign breast mass is to rule out a malignancy. Every woman's complaint should be taken seriously and given a complete evaluation. Therefore, the patient's risk of breast cancer needs to be assessed. Gender is the greatest risk factor for breast cancer. Only 1% of all breast cancers occur in men. This is likely related to the difference not only in estrogen, but also in progesterone. Age is another significant risk factor. A 30 year old woman has a 1:2,212 chance of being diagnosed with breast cancer. By the age of eighty, her chance increases to 1:8. The pathology of any previous biopsies should be obtained, especially if it was atypia, which as stated above, increases her risk from fourfold to ninefold. Information on previous radiation treatments should be obtained. Other important risk factors for breast cancer include prolonged exposure to estrogen, such as early menarche, late menopause, nulliparity, late parity (giving birth after the age of 35), or exogenous hormone treatment. Nulliparity increases a woman's risk by nearly 30%. There are few advantages to the use of combination hormonal replacement therapy (decreased osteoporosis, vaginal dryness, and hot flashes), and great disadvantages to hormonal therapy (increased risk of uterine cancer, cardiovascular side effects and breast cancer). It is imperative to obtain the family history, as familial carcinoma accounts for about 5–10% of all breast cancer. A woman's risk is increased if the affected family member is a first-degree relative (mother or sister). The risk increases from threefold to fourfold if the affected family member was premenopausal. An inquiry about family history of ovarian cancer should also be made. Women who are BRCA 1 or 2 have a 60–85% lifetime risk of breast cancer and a 40–65% of ovarian cancer risk. A woman's personal history of breast cancer is important to know because her risk of a new breast cancer continues to increase by approximately 1% per year.

Breast masses and tenderness are the most common physical complaints for which women seek medical attention for the breast. During the history and physical (H&P), note the presence and duration of any mass or change in the breast, any associated tenderness, any increase in size, and whether the mass changes with menses. Inquiries related to retraction and lymphadenopathy should be made. Questions on breast pain should include its relationship to cyclical changes, any changes with movement, whether the pain radiates, and if the patient has any bursitis-related symptoms. Details on dietary habits should be obtained, particularly including caffeine, chocolate, cheese, wine, and high fat meals. In addition, a history of cigarette smoking is important to note. These factors can be the source of breast pain and fibrocystic changes. An evaluation of any breast complaint should include questions about the nipple, such as scaliness, inversion/retraction, and discharge. Non-spontaneous nipple discharge that is green and nonbloody involving multiple ducts is often associated with benign conditions. When nipple discharge is from a single duct, spontaneous, grossly bloody, and/or clear, it warrants further evaluation. Ask whether the patient could be pregnant, which could be the reason for change in size of the breast or milky nipple discharge. Hormonal changes during pregnancy and/or lactation can be associated with bilateral bloody nipple discharge. Inquire about any recent trauma, which can be the source of a hematoma or fat necrosis that is presenting as a mass. However, caution the patient that breast cancer often presents with a recent trauma, perhaps because the trauma calls attention to the breast for examination.

Finally, be certain to ask whether the patient performs self breast examination (SBE), and whether she has noted any changes or differences. Review her technique to ensure she is performing it correctly. During the physical examination, be sure to explain to her what you are doing, so she can then incorporate these techniques into her own exam. During this part of patient education, teach the patient the mnemonic "BREAST" (Bumps, Retraction, Edema, Axillary mass, Skin changes, Tender/ Thickening), an acrostic for some signs and symptoms of breast cancer. In addition, emphasize that most breast cancers are asymptomatic, hence the importance of screening mammograms.

Physical Findings

When evaluating the breast, a thorough physical examination is necessary and should encompass the entire breast, chest wall, and the lymph nodes (axilla, supraclavicular, and cervical). Clinical breast examination depends on the technique and thoroughness of the examiner, and has a sensitivity of about 54% and specificity of 94%. The exam will be easiest the week after menses when the breast is not so tender and engorged. Physical exam begins with inspection of both breasts in the sitting and supine position. Compare both breasts for size, and remember that minor size differences are normal. Next, observe for any retraction of the skin, nipple, or breast itself. Retraction can be caused by tumor involvement of Cooper's ligaments. Also look for edema or peu d'orange in the skin, which is the orange peel-like appearance of the skin when there is tumor involvement of the dermal lymphatics (Fig. 1.1). Observe for any erythema or warmth of the breast. Mastitis and abscesses can present with these same signs, but it is important to remember that inflammatory breast cancer can also present in a similar fashion. Assess the nipple and areola for scaliness, which could indicate Paget's disease. Paget's disease occurs in about 1–2% of all women with breast cancer. Conversely, 90% of women who have Paget's disease have an underlying

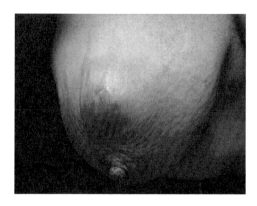

FIGURE 1.1. Peu d'orange of breast.

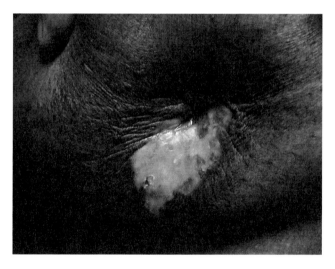

FIGURE 1.2. Scaliness and erosion of nipple secondary to Paget's disease.

breast cancer (Fig. 1.2). With the patient still in the upright position and with her arms relaxed, and from behind, palpate the axillary, subclavicular, and cervical lymph nodes, describing their location, consistency, and mobility.

Palpation of the breast should be done in the supine position with the ipsilateral arm behind the head, allowing the lateral quadrants and the tail of the breast to lie on the chest wall which makes palpation easier. Whether it is a concentric, radial, or lawn-mower pattern, palpation should proceed in an orderly fashion and encompass the entire anatomic boundaries of the breast. Extra attention should be given to any area of concern identified by the patient. The location of any discrete nodule or thickening should be described in terms of the distance from the nipple and the position of a clock face. The size, mobility, consistency, and borders of the mass should be described in the H&P. A dominant mass found on physical exam needs further investigation. The nipple-areola complex is gently squeezed to assess for any discharge and/or subareolar masses.

Breast pain could be due to referred pain from a myocardial infarction, hiatal hernia, disc disease, and cholelithiasis, so physical examination should also exclude these disorders. Chest wall pain could be musculoskeletal, thus assessment for trigger points should be complete. The most frequent cause of difficult-to-treat breast pain is bursitis. Breast pain associated with bursitis is important to diagnose, because it is the most often missed, and is simple to treat with physical therapy or trigger point injections.

Diagnostic Testing

Laboratory testing is rarely necessary during a breast work-up. However, for patients presenting with galactorrhea, prolactin, and thyroid levels may be necessary to rule out hypothyroidism, prolactinoma, and hyperprolactinemia. Because the sensitivity and specificity of clinical breast examination is not ideal, further diagnostic testing will be necessary and includes the "triple-negative test" (physical exam, imaging, and percutaneous biopsy). Patients may be safely followed if they have a "triple-negative test".

Diagnostic imaging includes mammography and ultrasound. Currently, mammography is the only imaging modality with proven effectiveness for breast cancer screening. Mammography has reduced mortality by 17% in women ages 40–49 and approximately 44% in women older than 50. However, it does have a false negative rate of 10–30%, and therefore, a biopsy should be performed on suspicious, palpable, or ultrasound-visible lesions, even with a negative mammogram.

Ultrasound has gained increased acceptance in the diagnosis and treatment of breast diseases (Fig. 1.3). Although not currently used for screening, ultrasound offers a significant advantage in the assessment of mammographic abnormalities or palpable lesions. It can be more beneficial in young high-risk women with dense breast, where mammography can be more difficult, and also in pregnant women to avoid the exposure to radiation. Ultrasound can also aid in the treatment of breast diseases. Most commonly, it can be used to localize lesions for office-based percutaneous biopsies and diagnosis

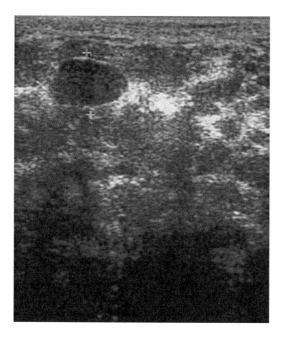

FIGURE 1.3. Mass on ultrasound.

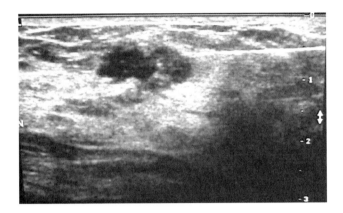

FIGURE 1.4. Core needle biopsy on ultrasound.

(Fig. 1.4). Frequently, it is used to guide needle or wire placement during needle-localization breast biopsies or to guide intraoperative removal of the US visible mass or the hematoma after a core biopsy of a non-visible lesion.

Breast MRI has been useful in evaluating breast lesions due to its sensitivity and specificity of 94–100% and 37–100%, respectively. MRI gives more detailed information on breast lesions; however, it is more expensive. MRI is covered by Medicare and private insurance if strict criteria are met. Clinical uses include assessing the success of neoadjuvant chemotherapy, detecting multicentric disease, and evaluating close or positive margins, as well as the evaluation of ruptured breast implants and axillary lymphadenopathy with an unknown primary.

Several different biopsy techniques will provide a diagnosis. The technique used will depend on the presentation of the lesion (palpable or nonpalpable), the patient, and the imaging modality available to guide the biopsy. These techniques include fine-needle aspiration (FNA), core needle biopsy (CNB), and open excisional biopsy (Figs. 1.5 and 1.6).

FNA is performed with a 22-gauge needle and yields cytological information, not histological, and results in insufficient data for diagnosis in up 36% of cases for nonpalpable lesions.

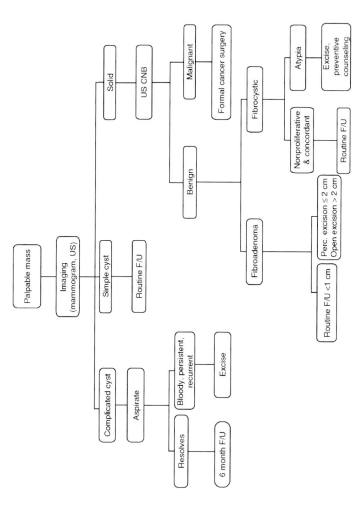

FIGURE 1.5. Treatment algorithm for palpable mass.

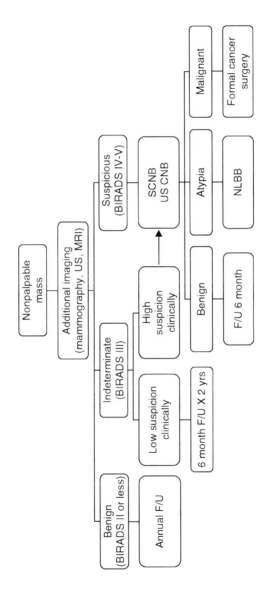

FIGURE 1.6. Treatment algorithm for non-palpable mass.

FNA may be advantageous only in patients with bleeding disorders. Core needle biopsy can be used for palpable lesions, or nonpalpable lesions under ultrasound or mammographic guidance. Needle sizes range from 14 gauge to 8 gauge, and when performed with vacuum-assisted devices, CNB provides large specimen sizes for good histological diagnosis (Fig. 1.4). Fibroadenomas can easily be diagnosed and removed by vacuum-assisted core needle biopsy in the clinic.

Mammographically guided or stereotactic core needle biopsy can be used for nonpalpable lesions, areas of architectural distortion, or suspicious microcalcifications found on mammogram. Patients who are not candidates for this procedure include those with lesions not clearly visualized in the stereotactic unit and those with very small breasts. Also, patients with a body weight too large for the stereotactic table, those who cannot lie prone, and those with arm movement limitations will not be candidates for this procedure.

Open excisional biopsy for diagnosis should be limited to nipple discharge, in which case the lesion is diagnosed and treated in the same setting. Excisional biopsy is indicated in patients who cannot undergo percutaneous or stereotactic core needle biopsy. It is also indicated when the core biopsy demonstrates atypia or is non-concordant. For microcalcifications or nonpalpable lesions, needle localization can be used to guide the excision. Both procedures are done in the operating room, with anesthesia ranging from local to general. Studies have shown that open excisional biopsy not only is more costly, but also increases the time to complete surgery and the need for repeated surgery.

Selected Readings

Bland K, Copeland E (2004) The breast: comprehensive management of benign and malignant disorders, 3rd edn. W.B. Saunders, St. Louis, MO

Hartmann LC, Sellers TA, Frost MH, et al. (2005) Benign breast disease and the risk of breast cancer. N Engl J Med 353:229–237

Harms SE (1998) Integration of breast magnetic resonance imaging with breast cancer treatment. Top Magn Reson Imaging 9:79

Klimberg VS (2004) Nipple discharge. In: Norton L Surgical decision making, 5th edn. Elsevier/Saunders, Philadelphia

Santen RJ, Mansel R (2005) Current concepts: benign breast disorders. N Engl J Med 353:275–285

Silva OE, Zurrida S (2003) Breast cancer: a practical guide. Elsevier Science, Oxford

2
Malignant Breast Disease: Diagnosis and Assessment

Nimmi Arora and Rache M. Simmons

Pearls and Pitfalls

- Screening mammography has allowed for earlier detection of breast cancer.
- Image-guided biopsy assists in the diagnosis of breast cancer.
- Infiltrating ductal carcinoma is the most common breast malignancy.
- Prognosis is based on stage at diagnosis.
- Breast-conserving surgery (lumpectomy) has become the treatment of choice for most patients.
- Whole-breast or partial-breast radiation treatment is used as an adjunct to breast-conserving surgery.
- Modified radical mastectomy or total mastectomy is used for large or diffuse breast cancer.
- Skin-sparing mastectomy allows for superior cosmesis.
- Breast reconstruction is encouraged after mastectomy.
- Sentinel lymph node biopsy may be used in place of axillary dissection to determine the presence of axillary metastasis for early-stage tumors without clinically suspicious nodes (cN0 axilla). If positive, a complete dissection should be performed in most breast cancer patients.
- Adjuvant hormone therapy for receptor-positive tumors has been shown to increase overall survival.
- Adjuvant chemotherapy for node-positive or large tumors has been shown to increase survival.

K.I. Bland et al. (eds.), *Surgery in Breast Cancer and Melanoma*, DOI 10.1007/978-1-84996-435-7_2,
© Springer-Verlag London Limited 2011

- Neoadjuvant chemotherapy can successfully downstage tumors, making them amenable for breast-conserving surgery.

Epidemiology

Breast cancer is the most common cancer in women worldwide. Globally, approximately one-quarter of female cancers are breast cancers and over one million women a year are diagnosed with the disease. Caucasian women of higher socioeconomic background in industrialized countries have the highest risk of developing breast cancer, whereas Asian and African races have a lower incidence of breast cancer. Geographically, the United States, the United Kingdom, Denmark, and New Zealand have some of the highest rates of breast cancer, while Japan, Thailand, Nigeria, and India have significantly lower rates. In the United States alone, one in eight women will be diagnosed with breast cancer in their lifetime.

Breast cancer continues to be the leading cause of cancer-related death in women ages 40–59, representing 14% of all deaths due to cancer in women worldwide and over 400,000 deaths in women per year. The National Cancer Institute data from the Surveillance, Epidemiology, and End Results (SEER) program during 1998–2002 reported that the age-adjusted incidence rate of breast cancer in the United States was 134.4 per 100,000 women per year, which was higher in Caucasians than in African-Americans. The age-adjusted death rate was 26.4 per 100,000 women per year, which was higher in African-Americans (at 34.7 per 100 K) than in Caucasians (at 25.9 per 100 K). The increase in mortality among African-American women is possibly attributed to a later stage of detection and more aggressive disease in this population.

Risk Factors

The most obvious, non-modifiable risk factors for breast cancer are age over 50 and female gender. This is followed by genetic factors – BRCA-1 and BRCA-2 – that are accountable for up to 10% of breast cancer cases in developed countries. Other risk factors include family history without documented BRCA mutation, personal history of breast cancer, prior breast biopsy revealing hyperplasia, LCIS or radial scars, and Caucasian race. Additional risk factors mostly seem to involve the increase in lifetime exposure to endogenous estrogens. This includes menarche before age 12, menopause after age 55, nulliparity, and first pregnancy after age 30, all of which cause an approximately twofold increase in the risk of breast cancer. Early pregnancy and early bilateral oophorectomy, on the other hand, have protective effects against breast cancer. Prior chest radiation therapy is also a risk factor, as in the example of mantle radiation for Hodgkin's lymphoma. While still controversial, exogenous hormone use may lend to a slight elevation in the risk of breast cancer, especially with longer duration of use. Alcohol consumption, obesity, and a sedentary lifestyle may also be risk factors.

Clinical Presentation

Routine screening mammography has allowed for early detection of most breast cancers prior to the development of any symptoms. Breast cancer can appear on mammography as a spiculated mass, an asymmetric density, a cluster of pleomorphic calcifications in ductal or segmental distribution, diffuse calcification, or a combination of these (see Figs. 2.1 and 2.2). When present, the most common clinical presentation of breast cancer is a palpable mass. The mass is usually painless, firm, and fixed. Additional findings associated with malignancy are skin or nipple retraction and bloody or serous nipple discharge. Scaling and an eczema-like rash of the nipple may indicate Paget's disease. Edema of the breast skin, or peau d'orange (resembling orange peel), often is due to inflammatory carcinoma or extensive axillary nodal disease, causing lymphatic obstruction. Typically, inflammatory carcinoma has associated erythema as well.

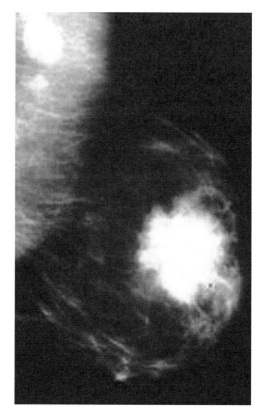

FIGURE 2.1. Mammogram of a large spiculated breast mass (Courtesy of Dr. Ruth Rosenblatt, Professor of Radiology, Weill Medical College of Cornell University).

Diagnosis

The American Cancer Society guidelines for breast cancer screening recommend annual mammograms for women beginning at the age of 40. In addition, clinical breast exams are recommended for women in their 20s and 30s every 3 years, and then annually at the age of 40. These guidelines have led to an earlier stage of detection of most breast cancers and, as a consequence, a significant decrease in mortality – as much as 32%.

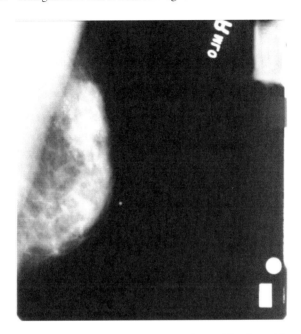

FIGURE 2.2. Mammogram of plesiomorphic calcifications (Courtesy of Dr. Ruth Rosenblatt).

In women with dense breast tissue, ultrasound may be more useful in detecting a suspicious lesion, as it can more readily discern cystic from solid lesions. Ultrasound can also be useful in defining a suspicious focus seen on mammography. MRI has become more commonly used in the detection of breast cancer as it has the highest sensitivity of all modalities. It is a useful adjunct to mammography, and can help better detect disease in patients with breast implants. In addition, MRI can be useful in detecting early stage cancers in high-risk patients such as those with a strong genetic predisposition or with prior chest radiation. Another use of MRI is to determine extent of disease (multi-focality) and whether a patient may undergo successful breast conservation surgery.

Once there is a suspicion of cancer based on either clinical breast exam or one of the imaging modalities or both, a biopsy should be performed to make a diagnosis. Since the majority of lesions are nonpalpable, image guidance is usually required. Ultrasound or mammography can be used for stereotactic or sonographic localization of a suspicious lesion. Fine needle aspiration (FNA) or core needle biopsy can then be performed with image guidance for nonpalpable lesions or without imaging for palpable lesions. Core needle biopsy is preferred over FNA since it provides more tissue and can evaluate histologic architecture. Often a core biopsy can distinguish the presence of invasion, histologic grade, and receptor status of a tumor. Excisional biopsy can also be done to diagnose a suspicious breast lesion. This can be performed with preoperative or intraoperative needle sonographic or mammographic localization if a lesion is nonpalpable. Using imaging, a wire is guided to the suspicious location within the breast. The wire facilitates the surgeon in accurately removing the area of the breast under question.

Pathology of Malignancy

The most common type of malignant breast cancer is infiltrating ductal carcinoma (IFDC), accounting for about 85% of all cancers. This tumor arises from and invades the walls of the ducts. It is often a solid tumor and can present as a hard mass on clinical exam. The prognosis for IFDC is dependent upon stage of diagnosis. Subtypes of IFDC are categorized by the prominent histologic features (see Fig. 2.3). Tubular carcinoma is one subtype with tubular structures, and mucinous carcinoma is another subtype characterized by a gelatinous matrix with slow-growing clusters of cells. Each of these subtypes represent about 2–3% of IFDC. Medullary carcinoma represents about 5% of IFDC and is distinguished by its large sheets of cells, often associated with hemorrhage or necrosis. Papillary carcinoma is another variant that can be intracystic and can present with serous or bloody nipple discharge.

Infiltrating lobular carcinoma (IFLC) represents another 15% of invasive breast cancer. It arises from the lobules of the breast. Clinically, IFLC can be difficult to diagnose. Often the clinical presentation is only a vague indistinct thickening. This is likely due to its histology of single-file arrangement of cells that can escape detection on both physical exam and mammography

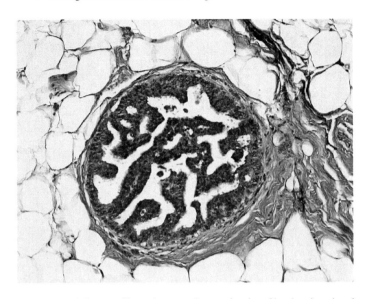

FIGURE 2.3. Micropapillary duct carcinoma in situ: Slender fronds of micropapillary ductal carcinoma in situ are present within a duct. The nuclear grade of the monotonous tumor cells is intermediate. The in situ carcinoma extends within 1 mm of the inked margin of resection (H&E stain) (Courtesy of Dr. Syed Hoda, Professor of Clinical Pathology, Weill Medical College of Cornell University).

(see Fig. 2.4). The prognosis is similar to IFDC and is based upon stage of diagnosis. Some tumors will take on mixed ductal and lobular features and will be described as such.

Inflammatory carcinoma is diagnosed clinically when tumor cells of the breast block lymphatic channels and cause the affected breast to be erythematous, edematous, warm, indurated, and classically with a peau d'orange appearance. This poorly differentiated tumor is diagnosed when evidence of dermal lymphatic involvement is present. This is typically diagnosed histologically from a punch skin biopsy. Metastasis to axillary lymph nodes is common in these patients at initial presentation. Patients with inflammatory carcinoma have an extremely poor prognosis, and treatment consists of combination therapy usually including neoadjuvant chemotherapy followed by mastectomy and postoperative chest wall radiation therapy.

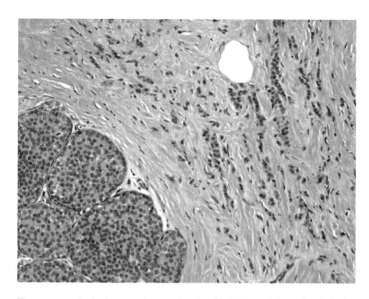

FIGURE 2.4. Lobular carcinoma in situ (LCIS) and invasive lobular carcinoma: Lobular carcinoma in situ is characterized by neoplastic proliferation of monotonous cells that distend and distort the lobules. Invasive lobular carcinoma shows characteristic "indian filing" architectural pattern amidst dense stromal fibrosis? (H&E stain) (Courtesy of Dr. Syed Hoda).

Paget's disease is an uncommon form of breast cancer that presents as scaling or crusting of the nipple. Underlying breast cancer, usually IFDC, is almost always associated with this presentation. Diagnosis is made by a nipple skin biopsy that reveals Pagetoid cells. The underlying cancer determines treatment and prognosis.

Other rare forms of breast cancer are malignant phyllodes tumors, angiosarcomas, lymphomas, and squamous cell carcinomas. Malignant phyllodes tumors require wide local excision for treatment. These tumors behave clinically as a sarcoma, with typical metastasis to the lungs rather than the axilla.

Thus axillary dissection is not beneficial in patients with malignant phyllodes tumors. Angiosarcomas are rare and are associated with previous radiation therapy. They tend to behave aggressively and are treated with excision, often requiring mastectomy and adjuvant chemotherapy. Lymphomas and squamous cell carcinomas are treated as they are in other parts of the body.

Staging

Breast cancers are classified using the American Joint Committee on Cancer (AJCC) system that describes the tumor (T), nodal status (N), and the presence of metastasis (M) (Table 2.1). This classification allows for breast cancers to be sorted into stages (Table 2.2) that can then predict relapse rates and form the basis for treatment algorithms. The current AJCC system includes the number of malignant regional lymph nodes as criteria for staging.

In addition to the TNM staging system, other prognostic factors useful in predicting the behavior of some breast cancers include hormone receptor status and histologic grade. The presence of hormone receptors affect prognosis. Patients diagnosed with invasive breast cancer whose tumors are positive for either estrogen receptor (ER), progesterone receptor (PR), or both have a significantly better survival overall, with the best survival in both ER-positive and PR-positive cancers. Histologic grade, which is determined by cellular architecture, nuclear differentiation, and mitotic rate, also predicts time to recurrence and survival.

Bone marrow micrometastases can be identified via bone marrow aspiration and have been shown to predict distant recurrence and prognosis. Other markers, such as HER2/neu (an epithelial growth factor) and cathepsin D (an estrogen-induced lysosomal protease), may be negative prognostic indicators of disease-free survival and overall survival.

Treatment

Surgical Management of Breast Cancer

Surgical treatment of breast cancer is based on stage of disease. Fifty years ago, the radical mastectomy was the mainstay of treatment. To date, numerous trials have demonstrated that

TABLE 2.1. TNM classification for breast cancer from the AJCC cancer staging manual, 6th edition.

Primary tumor (T)

TX	Primary tumor cannot be assessed
T0	No evidence of primary tumor
Tis	Carcinoma in situ
Tis (DCIS)	Ductal carcinoma in situ
Tis (LCIS)	Lobular carcinoma in situ
Tis (Paget)	Paget's disease of the nipple with no tumor (Paget's disease associated with a tumor is classified according to the size of the tumor)
T1	Tumor $\leq$ 2 cm in greatest dimension
T1mic	Microinvasion $\leq$ 0.1 cm in greatest dimension
T1a	Tumor > 0.1 cm but $\leq$ 0.5 cm in greatest dimension
T1b	Tumor > 0.5 cm but $\leq$ 1 cm in greatest dimension
T1c	Tumor > 1 cm but $\leq$ 2 cm in greatest dimension
T2	Tumor > 2 cm but $\leq$ 5 cm in greatest dimension
T3	Tumor > 5 cm in greatest dimension
T4	Tumor of any size with direct extension to chest wall or skin, only as described below
T4a	Extension to chest wall, not including pectoralis muscle
T4b	Edema (including peau d'orange) or ulceration of the skin of the breast, or satellite skin nodules confined to the same breast
T4c	Both T4a and T4b
T4d	Inflammatory carcinoma

Regional lymph nodes (N)

NX	Regional lymph nodes cannot be assessed (e.g., previously removed)
N0	No regional lymph node metastasis
N1	Metastasis in movable ipsilateral axillary lymph node(s)

(continued)

TABLE 2.1. (continued)

N2	Metastasis in ipsilateral axillary lymph nodes fixed or matted, or in clinically apparent[a] ipsilateral internal mammary nodes in the absence of clinically evident axillary lymph node metastasis
N2a	Metastasis in ipsilateral axillary lymph nodes fixed to one another (matted) or to other structures
N2b	Metastasis only in clinically apparent[a] ipsilateral internal mammary nodes and in the absence of clinically evident axillary lymph node metastasis
N3	Metastasis in ipsilateral infraclavicular lymph node(s), or in clinically apparent[a] ipsilateral internal mammary lymph node(s) and in the presence of clinically evident axillary lymph node metastasis; metastasis in ipsilateral supraclavicular lymph node(s) with or without axillary or internal mammary lymph node involvement
N3a	Metastasis in ipsilateral infraclavicular lymph node(s) and axillary lymph node(s)
N3b	Metastasis in ipsilateral internal mammary lymph node(s) and axillary lymph node(s)
N3c	Metastasis in ipsilateral supraclavicular lymph node(s)

Regional lymph nodes (pN)[b]

pNX	Regional lymph nodes cannot be assessed (e.g., previously removed or not removed for pathologic study)
pN0	No regional lymph node metastasis histologically, no additional examination for isolated tumor cells[c]
pN0(i–)	No regional lymph node metastasis histologically, negative immunohistochemical staining
pN0(i+)	Isolated tumor cells identified histologically or by positive immunohistochemical staining, no cluster > 0.2 mm[d]
pN0(mol–)	No regional lymph-node metastasis histologically, negative molecular findings (RT-PCR)[e]
	No regional lymph-node metastasis histologically, positive molecular findings (RT-PCR)[e]

(continued)

TABLE 2.1. (continued)

pN1	Metastasis in one to three axillary lymph nodes, and/or in internal mammary nodes with microscopic disease detected by sentinel lymph node dissection but not clinically apparent[a]
pN1mi	Micrometastasis (>0.2 mm, none > 2.0 mm)
pN1a	Metastasis in 1–3 axillary lymph nodes
pN1b	Metastasis in internal mammary nodes with microscopic disease detected by sentinel lymph node dissection but not clinically apparent[a]
pN1c	Metastasis in one to three axillary lymph nodes[f] and in internal mammary lymph nodes with microscopic disease detected by sentinel lymph-node dissection but not clinically apparent[a]
pN2	Metastasis in four to nine axillary lymph nodes, or in clinically apparent[a] internal mammary lymph nodes in the absence of axillary lymph node metastasis
pN2a	Metastasis in four to nine axillary lymph nodes (at least one tumor deposit > 2 mm)
pN2b	Metastasis in clinically apparent[a] internal mammary lymph nodes in the absence of axillary lymph node metastasis
pN3	Metastasis in 10 or more axillary lymph nodes, or in infraclavicular lymph nodes, or in clinically apparent[a] ipsilateral internal mammary lymph nodes in the presence of one or more positive axillary lymph nodes; or in more than three axillary lymph nodes with clinically negative microscopic metastasis in internal mammary lymph nodes; or in ipsilateral supraclavicular lymph nodes
pN3a	Metastasis in 10 or more axillary lymph nodes (at least one tumor deposit > 2 mm), or metastasis to the infraclavicular lymph nodes
pN3b	Metastasis in clinically apparent[a] ipsilateral internal mammary lymph nodes in the presence of one or more positive axillary lymph nodes; or in more than three lymph nodes with microscopic disease detected by sentinel lymph axillary lymph nodes and in internal mammary node dissection but not clinically apparent[a]
pN3c	Metastasis in ipsilateral supraclavicular lymph nodes

(continued)

TABLE 2.1. (continued)

Distant metastasis (M)

MX	Distant metastasis cannot be assessed
M0	No distant metastasis
M1	Distant metastasis

[a] *Clinically apparent is defined as detected by imaging studies (excluding lymphoscintigraphy) or by clinical examination.*

[b] *Classification is based on axillary lymph node dissection with or without sentinel lymph node dissection. Classification based solely on sentinel lymph node dissection without subsequent axillary lymph node dissection is designated (sn) for "sentinel node," such as pN0 (i+) (sn).*

[c] *Isolated tumor cells are defined as single tumor cells or small cell clusters 0.2 mm, usually detected only by immunohistochemical or molecular methods but which may be verified on hematoxylin and eosin stains. Isolated tumor cells do not usually show evidence of metastatic activity (e.g., proliferation or stromal reaction).*

[d] *Definition of (i+) was adapted in 2003 in order to be consistent with the updated International Union Against Cancer (UICC) classification.*

[e] *RT-PCR: reverse transcriptase/polymerase chain reaction.*

[f] *If associated with more than three positive axillary lymph nodes, the internal mammary nodes are classified as pN3b to reflect increased tumor burden.*

breast conservation surgery (BCS) along with radiation therapy allows equal survival to mastectomy. Thus breast conservation has largely replaced the mastectomy for most women currently diagnosed with breast cancer.

Radical mastectomy involves en bloc resection of the breast, overlying skin, nipple, pectoral muscles, and axillary contents. Although it is rarely required, this surgical option can offer palliative treatment for disease that extends into the chest wall. The modified radical mastectomy (MRM) has largely replaced the radical mastectomy, and includes the removal of the breast and axillary contents while preserving the pectoral muscles. There is no difference between the two in overall survival. For patients with negative axillary lymph nodes, total mastectomy with sentinel node biopsy is often performed instead of MRM. Both the MRM and the total mastectomy can be performed using a skin-sparing technique

TABLE 2.2. TNM stage grouping.

Stage 0	Tis	N0	M0
Stage I	T1a	N0	M0
Stage IIA	T0	N1	M0
	T1a	N1	M0
	T2	N0	M0
Stage IIB	T2	N1	M0
	T3	N0	M0
Stage IIIA	T0	N2	M0
	T1[a]	N2	M0
	T2	N2	M0
	T3	N1	M0
	T3	N2	M0
Stage IIIB	T4	N0	M0
	T4	N1	M0
	T4	N2	M0
Stage IIIC	Any T	N3	M0
Stage IV	Any T	Any N	M1

[a]T1 includes T1mic.

in selected breast cancer patients. Skin-sparing mastectomy preserves the skin envelope of the breast allowing for improved cosmesis for reconstruction. This is contraindicated in inflammatory breast cancer and other cases in which the overlying breast skin is extensively involved with cancer.

Breast reconstruction is recommended for any woman undergoing mastectomy and can be performed either immediately or in a delayed fashion. Several forms of reconstruction exist. A tissue expander and breast implant is one in which expansion of the pectoralis muscles is performed for several weeks to allow for placement of a permanent saline or silicone implant. Tissue flap reconstructions are other alternatives, with the most common of these being the transverse rectus abdominis myocutaneous (TRAM) flap. This involves transferring skin, fat, muscle, and blood supply from the abdomen to create a new breast.

Breast conservation surgery includes local excision (lumpectomy, quadrantectomy, segmental resection, partial mastectomy) with microscopically negative margins. The National Surgical Adjuvant Breast and Bowel Project (NSABP) has conducted numerous randomized controlled trials to compare treatment modalities. The NSABP B-06 protocol compared lumpectomy and axillary node dissection with or without breast radiation to total mastectomy and found that there was no significant difference in overall survival between the groups. An earlier study from Milan also established that quadrantectomy with axillary dissection and radiation for tumors less than 2 cm without clinically suspicious axillary nodes showed no difference in survival when compared to radical mastectomy.

For most patients with invasive or non-invasive disease, lumpectomy with radiation has been shown to have lower local recurrence rates compared to lumpectomy alone. After 20 years of follow-up, local recurrence in lumpectomy with radiation was 14.3%, while lumpectomy alone was 39.2% ($P < 0.001$).

There are data to suggest that in select patients with only ductal carcinoma in situ (DCIS) and low risk of recurrence, radiation can be omitted without increased risk of local recurrence. These women must meet the criteria of low-grade DCIS and clean surgical margins of 10 mm or more.

BCS, is not, although, the appropriate treatment for every patient with breast cancer. BCS is contraindicated in women with more than one ipsilateral tumor in different breast quadrants, diffuse disease as demonstrated by large areas of mammographic calcifications, or large tumor size. Patients with tumors greater than 5 cm are often stated as inappropriate candidates for BCS, although this really depends upon the ratio of resection relative to the size of the treated breast. Patients with contraindications for radiation therapy such as prior chest radiation therapy, pregnancy, and previous BCS, would also be considered inappropriate candidates for BCS. Failed BCS may also be an indication for mastectomy.

Breast cancer is thought to spread first to the regional axillary lymph nodes; therefore the status of these lymph nodes gives important information regarding staging, prognosis, and recommendations for therapy. Traditionally all patients diagnosed with breast cancer would undergo an axillary dissection to evaluate the lymph node status. This involves removal of 10–30 lymph nodes from the axilla. The potential complications of this operation include ipsilateral arm lymphedema, upper arm numbness, seroma formation, and increased risk of future arm infections. An alternative to an axillary lymph node dissection (ALND) is a sentinel lymph node biopsy (SLNB). The sentinel lymph node is the first node or nodes in the axillary chain that receive drainage from the breast. These sentinel nodes are therefore the most likely nodes to be affected by metastasis if it has occurred. The technique of SLNB requires injection of isosulfan or methylene blue dye and/or a radioactive isotope into the affected breast. These markers are taken up in the lymphatic system just as a malignant cell would be and identifies the sentinel nodes. SLNB has proven to be accurate in identifying patients with axillary metastases in breast cancer patients, and it minimizes the complications of the more invasive ALND. There are multiple studies in the literature demonstrating that if a SLN is negative for metastatic disease, then the remaining axillary nodes are negative as well, and additional axillary dissection is not warranted. Also the exceedingly low rate of reported axillary recurrences in SLN-negative patients supports the clinical efficacy of SLNB.

In general, for patients with histologically H&E positive SLN, completion axillary dissection is recommended. However, it is debatable whether all patients with positive SLN are justified in having further axillary dissection. It has been documented that in 50–70% of patients, the SLN is the only positive node. The removal of additional negative axillary lymph nodes offers no clinical advantage and only increases potential morbidity. Most surgeons today use completion axillary dissection selectively. Informational tools such as nomograms help surgeons determine each patient's risk of additional positive remaining axillary nodes, and take into account tumor type, nuclear grade, lymphovascular invasion, multifocality of the primary tumor, estrogen-receptor status, number of positive SLN, pathological size, and the method of detection of SLN metastases. This information can be utilized in patient – surgeon discussions regarding further axillary dissection on an individual basis.

One topic on which there is considerable debate is the clinical significance of SLN micrometastases. In contrast to traditional ALND, SLNB affords the opportunity to extensively evaluate limited axillary nodes with more detailed analysis. Typically each SLN will be evaluated by serial sectioning with H&E, and at many institutions, additional immunohistochemistry (IHC) testing for the presence of metastatic disease is based on the presence of cytokeratin. In particular, IHC is able to identify micrometastases (0.2–2 mm) and isolated cancer cells (<0.2 mm), though the therapeutic implications of these results are currently unknown.

Among those patients with T1–3 invasive breast cancer, there are relative contraindications that may preclude some women as candidates for SLNB. Clinical situations that cause concern about the accuracy of SLNB due to the potential disruption of lymphatic drainage include extensive ipsilateral axillary surgery, previous SLNB/ALND, extensive upper outer quadrant resection, and ipsilateral radiation therapy. There are series in the literature showing that in all situations described above and even in the setting of a previous SLNB or ALND, a SLNB can be attempted. The likelihood of identification of SLN can be less in these settings, but if a definite SLN is identified, results have been shown to be reliable. Clinically palpable lymph nodes or those suspicious on ultrasound warrant further investigation via fine needle aspiration (FNA). If the FNA is found to be positive, this indicates ALND without SLNB. If negative, these nodes should be considered indeterminate and evaluated by SLNB. It has been shown that clinically suspicious lymph nodes often do not represent metastatic disease and may instead represent benign reactive lymph nodes, especially in the setting of a diagnostic core biopsy.

Adjuvant Therapy

Adjuvant therapy for breast cancer consists of radiation therapy, chemotherapy, and hormonal therapy. Adjuvant therapy has significantly improved survival and is considered standard for all patients with node-positive disease.

Radiation therapy is used for all women after lumpectomy for invasive cancer. As discussed earlier, this has significantly increased disease-free survival. Standard treatment involves external beam radiation to the whole breast daily for a period of about 6 weeks. Accelerated partial breast irradiation offers localized radiation therapy to the lumpectomy site in abbreviated time compared to conventional whole breast external beam radiation. Trials are ongoing as to the efficacy of accelerated partial breast radiation compared to whole breast irradiation.

Systemic adjuvant chemotherapy has become a mainstay of treatment for patients with node-positive breast cancer and those tumors where the invasive component measures greater than 1 cm. In these settings, chemotherapy offers patients a significant survival advantage. Women with other high risk factors may also be offered chemotherapy based on tumor characteristics. In general, multiple drug combinations are more effective than single-agent therapy.

Neoadjuvant chemotherapy, or preoperative chemotherapy, has been useful in downstaging tumors. Especially in patients who would not be candidates for lumpectomy, neoadjuvant chemotherapy can reduce the size of many of these tumors and make them amenable to BCS. The NSABP protocol B-18 showed no difference in overall survival or disease-free survival in patients given neoadjuvant chemotherapy compared to postoperative chemotherapy.

Hormonal therapy for women with ER-positive breast cancers has also proven to give a survival benefit and has become a standard part of adjuvant therapy. Selective Estrogen Receptor Modulators (SERMs) such as tamoxifen are used in combination with radiation therapy and chemotherapy to improve survival. Tamoxifen significantly improves both disease-free and overall survival when compared to placebo after surgery for breast cancer. As seen in the NSABP B-14 study, recurrence-free survival in patients treated with tamoxifen was 78% compared to only 65% in those receiving placebo. In addition, tamoxifen reduces the incidence of contralateral breast cancer. Survival is improved even more when tamoxifen is given in addition to chemotherapy for women < 60 years of age. Tamoxifen is not beneficial as adjuvant treatment for ER-negative invasive breast cancers. Optimal duration of treatment with tamoxifen is approximately 5 years for node-negative patients, and given after 5 years in node-positive patients on individual basis. Side effects include menopausal symptoms such as hot flashes, increased risk of uterine tumors, and increased risk of thrombotic events.

Aromatase inhibitors have also been shown to play a role in adjuvant therapy for hormone receptor-positive tumors. Recent studies, such as the ATAC trial, have shown that aromatase inhibitors such as anastrozole or letrozole may be more beneficial with fewer side effects than tamoxifen. Optimal duration and timing of treatment with aromatase inhibitors is still being investigated. Molecular targeted adjuvant therapy is also an active area of research in breast cancer. Trastuzumab, an antiHER2 antibody, has shown some success, though safety and efficacy are yet to be determined.

Follow-up

The majority of breast cancer recurrences occur within the first 3 years of treatment. As such, patients should follow-up for physical exams every 3–6 months for the first 3 years, every 6–12 months for the following 2 years, and then annually thereafter. Annual mammograms should also be continued on contralateral breasts every 6 months for 2 years, then annually for the ipsilateral breast treated with BCS. Unless indicated from clinical symptoms or physical exam, bone scans and CT scans are not routinely used in follow-up. Annual pelvic exams with ultrasound to evaluate uterine wall thickness should be done for any patient taking tamoxifen as the risk of endometrial cancer is increased.

Special Topics: Male Breast Cancer

Breast cancer in men accounts for less than 1% on all breast cancer diagnosed. Risk factors include older age, family history of breast cancer, and radiation exposure. Estrogen administration or diseases that expose men to higher levels of estrogen, such as liver failure or Klinefelter's syndrome, may also predispose men to a higher risk of breast cancer. Diagnosis is often delayed due to lack of screening. Patients typically present with a firm, painless, subareolar mass. Mammography and/or ultrasound can be useful in distinguishing gynecomastia from malignancy. Biopsies should be performed on all suspicious lesions. As with women, infiltrating ductal carcinoma is the most common tumor type. Treatment of male breast cancer consists of mastectomy with either SLNB or axillary dissection. Prognosis is identical to female breast cancer as based upon stage of diagnosis. Adjuvant therapy is determined by similar criteria used in female breast cancer. The majority of male breast cancers are estrogen receptor positive, and tamoxifen is typically offered in the adjuvant setting.

Special Topics: Breast Cancer in Pregnancy

Breast cancer is the most common cancer in pregnant women, accounting for 2% of all breast cancers. Delays in diagnosis are due to the difficulty of examining the breasts of pregnant women as they are naturally tender and engorged, as well as the fact that mammography is not performed while pregnant. Ultrasound should be used to evaluate suspicious findings. Biopsies should be performed on all lesions under question in pregnant patients. Since radiation is contraindicated in pregnancy, mastectomy is the treatment of choice unless the diagnosis is late in pregnancy and radiation can be safely deferred until delivery. The safety of SLNB in pregnancy is controversial. Adjuvant chemotherapy, if indicated, can be given during the second and third trimesters.

Special Topics: Chemoprevention

Studies have shown that women at high risk of breast cancer can lower their risk by taking either tamoxifen or raloxifene for 5 years. The NSABP P-1 trial showed a decrease in the incidence of ER-positive breast cancer by almost 50%. The STAR trial compared tamoxifen and raloxifene to each other and found that raloxifene is not only as effective as tamoxifen in reducing the risk of breast cancer, but it also has a statistically significant lower risk of uterine cancer than tamoxifen.

The potential harmful side effects of SERMs such as thromboembolic events, endometrial cancer, and symptomatic effects (hot flashes), must be weighed against the benefits of these drugs on an individual basis. Those patients at highest risk of developing breast cancer and at lower risks for serious side effects would likely benefit the most from chemoprevention.

Selected Readings

ATAC Trialists' Group (2005) Results of the ATAC (Arimidex, Tamoxifen, Alone or in Combination) trial after completion of 5 years' adjuvant treatment for breast cancer. Lancet 365:60–62

Braun S, Vogl FD, Naume B, et al. (2005) A pooled analysis of bone marrow micrometastasis in breast cancer. N Engl J Med 353:793–802

Fisher B, Costantino J, Redmond C, et al. (1989) A randomized clinical trial evaluating tamoxifen in the treatment of patients with node-negative breast cancer who have estrogen-receptor positive tumors. N Engl J Med 320:479–484

Fisher B, Costantino JP, Wickerham DL, et al. (1998) Tamoxifen for prevention of breast cancer: report of the National Surgical Adjuvant Breast and Bowel Project P-1 Study. J Natl Cancer Inst 90:1371–1388

Fisher ER, Anderson S, Redmond C, Fisher B (1993) Pathologic findings from the National Surgical Adjuvant Breast Project protocol B-06. 10-year pathologic and clinical prognostic discriminants. Cancer 71:2507–2514

Silverstein MJ (2003) An argument against routine use of radiotherapy for ductal carcinoma in situ. Oncology (Williston Park) 17:1511–1533

Simmons RM, Fish SK, Gayle L, et al. (1999) Local and distant recurrence rates in skin-sparing mastectomies compared with non-skin-sparing mastectomies. Ann Surg Oncol 6:676–681

Zee Van KJ, Manasseh DM, Bevilacqua JL, et al. (2003) A nomogram for predicting the likelihood of additional nodal metastases in breast cancer patients with a positive sentinel node biopsy. Ann Surg Oncol 10:1140–1151

Vogel VG, Costantino JP, Wickerham DL, et al. (2006) (NSABP). Effects of tamoxifen vs raloxifene on the risk of developing invasive breast cancer and other disease outcomes: the NSABP Study of Tamoxifen and Raloxifene (STAR) P-2 trial. JAMA 295:2727–2741

Wolmark N, Wang J, Mamounas E, et al. (2001) Preoperative chemotherapy in patients with operable breast cancer: nine-year results from National Surgical Adjuvant Breast and Bowel Project B-18. J Natl Cancer Inst Monogr (30):96–102

3

High Risk Indicators: Microscopic Lesions, Personal and Family History, Assessment, and Management

Susan W. Caro and David L. Page

Pearls and Pitfalls

- It is possible to identify women at increased risk of developing breast cancer, and to offer increased surveillance or measures to decrease risk for these women.
- Discussion of breast cancer risk should be done with care, with an appreciation of the complex concepts, imprecise nature of risk assessments, and an effort not to create undue anxiety and fear for the patient and her family.
- The most important risk factors for breast cancer include: female gender, advancing age, family history, increased mammographic density, and pathologic indicators of increased risk.
- Neither physiologic menopausal hormone replacement therapy nor oral contraceptive use significantly alters breast cancer risk.
- Clinical testing is now commercially available for several breast cancer susceptibility genes, and is best offered by health care providers, including nurses and counselors, specially trained in cancer genetics.
- Women at increased risk of developing breast cancer may consider options of increasedsurveillance, risk-reducing medications, or surgeries.

Although breast cancer requires vigilance in screening in all women, we are able with some confidence to identify women at significantly increased risk of developing breast cancer.

K.I. Bland et al. (eds.), *Surgery in Breast Cancer and Melanoma*, DOI 10.1007/978-1-84996-435-7_3, © Springer-Verlag London Limited 2011

Identification of those at high risk provides the opportunity to offer women increased surveillance and measures to decrease risk.

Concepts of Risk

Health care providers must be cautious in explaining concepts of risk of breast cancer. As always in medicine, one must take into account the individual patient's ability to understand these often complex issues. With breast cancer, complexity is enhanced by common discussions in the lay press in which the news of the day may have little relevance in the background of information more relevant to the individual patient. A discussion of the concepts of risk is further clarified by beginning with the question, risk of what: The risk of developing breast cancer, the risk of dying of breast cancer, or the risk of having a proven inherited predisposition to breast cancer? A major part of the discussion must involve the denominator of the number of years at risk and the age of the patient. We are relieved that quoting of a lifetime risk is now unusual, as it does not relate well to an individual patient's understanding of their condition, and is a better indication of the burden of society of breast cancer and not an indication of individual risk. This must be understood to operate over a finite time from the age of assessment. Time periods of 10–15 years from indication of risk factors have been verified for similar women of similar ages. For example, a woman in her forties should not be overly concerned about management if there is an increased possibility of breast cancer occurring in her seventies.

Lifetime Risk

The lifetime risk for breast cancer for a given population is the risk of developing breast cancer during one's lifetime. This estimate is 1 in 8 for women in the United States, assuming that they are at risk for 90 years. The lifetime risk of dying of breast cancer is 1 in 28.

Relative Risk

Relative risk (RR) is a measure of the strength of a risk factor or condition and its association with cancer. Relative risk compares the risk of cancer in one group with the risk in a reference population, which is usually the general population, or a group without the specific risk factor. A relative risk of 1 means no difference between the two groups. A relative risk of 2 means that the risk of one group is twofold, or two times, the risk in the reference population. This can also be expressed as a 100% increase in risk. Risks of this nature, when reported in the media without an adequate explanation of what the term means, can be confusing and frightening for women. It is possible, however, to take a relative risk and use age-adjusted risks to determine risk estimates over specific time periods. For example: If one considers the relative risk of developing breast cancer to be 1.7 for women with a first-degree relative with breast cancer, the risk of developing breast cancer for a woman aged 40 years during her 40th year might increase from approximately 1 in 1,000 during that year to 1.7 in 1,000. An abstract or comparative risk is not useful clinically unless it can be placed in context for the individual woman being counseled.

Absolute Risk

Absolute risk (AR) is the risk of developing cancer over a specified time period. Estimates of absolute risk are based on age-adjusted risk over a specified time. That is, it is far more useful for a patient to know her own risk of developing breast cancer, AR, than to know how much more likely she is to develop breast cancer than some other woman (RR). Dupont and Plummer have developed software to help clinicians translate relative risks into absolute risks, and graphs demonstrating absolute risks that can be used to aid in applying RR information to the individual woman (see Dupont and Plummer, 1996; Dupont, 1989, and http://biostat.mc.vanderbilt. edu/twiki/bin/view/ Main/RelativeToAbsoluteRisks.

TABLE 3.1. Classification of breast cancer risk.

Slight or mild risk elevation	1.5–2 times comparison group
Moderate risk elevation	4–5 times comparison group
High risk elevation	9–11 times comparison group

Rationale: 10 times is about as great an elevation of risk as has been demonstrated to be reliably predicted in any group of women over a 10–15 year period (the range often chosen for counseling).

It is also important to consider what degree of risk is of clinical importance. What degree of risk might alter consideration of interventions for decreasing risk? In the authors' view, only a relative risk of 2, or one that is reliably determined to be at least double that of the general population, qualifies as a clinically meaningful, elevated risk (see Table 3.1).

Breast cancer is relatively common in women, accounting for approximately 30% of new cancer diagnoses each year in American women. The probability of developing cancer of any site for women in the United States from birth to death is 1 in 3. The often-quoted "lifetime risk" of developing breast cancer is 1 in 8, or 12%. The majority of women diagnosed have no significant identifiable risk factors. This is why screening of all women is so important.

Risk Factors for Breast Cancer

Female gender and advanced age are the most important elements in the risk of breast cancer. Breast cancer does occur in men, although it is much less common. Often cited hormonal factors that may be associated with an increased risk of breast cancer include early menarche, late menopause, nulliparity, and first childbirth after age 30. Lactation, early childbirth, and early menopause are associated with decreased risk. However, none of these factors alter risk by a significant amount, with less than 50% alteration of risk associated with any given factor in most reports. Mammographic increased density has been associated with increased risk, somewhat over double.

There is a vast amount of literature on diet, weight, exercise, and other lifestyle factors and breast cancer risk. Factors such as exercise have been demonstrated to be associated with a decrease in breast cancer risk, with weight gain and alcohol consumption associated with an increase in risk. None of these factors is associated with a clinically significant alteration in risk, in other words, a relative risk of greater than two. We have little knowledge of the interactions among specific risk factors except where such interactions have been studied specifically. Some of these have included the tissue-based assessment of risk (particularly the atypical hyperplasias), family history, and postmenopausal hormone replacement. However there is little synergy here, and risk associated with atypical hyperplasia remains unaltered by hormone replacement therapy and little altered by co-existing family history.

Age

Advancing age is a significant risk factor for breast cancer. Table 3.2 provides some age-adjusted risk estimates that are helpful in putting risk in perspective for the individual woman.

TABLE 3.2. Age and breast cancer (general female population, United States) (Adapted from Reis et al., 1999; Henderson, 1993; American Cancer Society, 2000; Feuer et al., 1993).

Possibility of developing breast cancer	Approximate age adjusted risk per year	
	Age	Risk during that year
Age 0–39 = 1 in 231 (0.43%)	30	1 in 5,000
Age 40–59 = 1 in 25 (4%)	40	1 in 1,000
	50	1 in 500
Age 60–79 = 1 in 15 (6.88%)	60	1 in 350
	70	1 in 270
Lifetime = 1 in 8 (12%)	80	1 in 250

TABLE 3.3. Age-specific probability of developing invasive breast carcinoma in 10-year intervals.

Current age in years	No increased risk	2 × Increased risk	4 × Increased risk
20	1 in 2,000	1 in 1,000	1 in 500
30	1 in 256	1 in 128	1 in 64
40	1 in 67	1 in 34	1 in 17
50	1 in 39	1 in 20	1 in 10
60	1 in 29	1 in 15	1 in 7

Another way of evaluating this parameter is by assessing the risk of developing breast cancer in specific time periods as shown in Table 3.3.

Family History

A family history of breast cancer has long been known to be associated with breast cancer risk. Women with a family history of breast or ovarian cancer may be at significantly increased risk for developing cancer. The family history is most important when it includes multiple family members, cancer diagnosed at younger ages, and bilateral or multiple cancer sites. Women who have a prior personal history of breast or ovarian cancer are also at increased risk.

Pathologic Indicators of Risk

Prior to delineation of specific pathologic indicators of increased risk for breast cancer in the 1980s, it was believed that women who had a history of prior benign breast biopsies had a 2–5 times greater risk of developing breast cancer. Since that time, many studies have defined the specific lesions of benign breast biopsies that are associated with increased risk and those that are not. The benign breast lesions and associated risks are listed in Table 3.4. It is important to recognize that breast cancer risk estimation is not a simple dichotomous "yes or no" determination. It is complex, with a broad range of magnitudes, and a range of weaker and stronger certainties.

As seen in Table 3.4, the pathologic findings associated with fibrocystic changes are not associated with significant elevations of risk. Although breast cysts in general are not

TABLE 3.4. Relative risk of invasive breast carcinoma based on the microscopic examination of otherwise benign breast tissue, usually at biopsy.

Slightly increased risk (1.5–2 times)

Women with the following lesions have a slightly increased risk for invasive breast carcinoma compared with women who have not had a breast biopsy, as well as women whose breast biopsies lack these lesions on microscopic examination:

Moderate or florid hyperplasia without atypia	Common
Fibroadenoma with complex features	Uncommon
Sclerosing adenosis	Relatively common
Solitary papilloma without coexistent atypical hyperplasia	Relatively common

Moderately increased risk (4.5–5.9 times)

Women with the following lesions have a moderately increased risk of invasive breast carcinoma compared with women who have not had a breast biopsy:

Atypical ductal hyperplasia (ADH)

Atypical lobular hyperplasia (ALH)

Focal ductal pattern atypia in appaloosas

Markedly increased risk (8–10 times)

Women with the following lesions have a high risk of invasive breast carcinoma compared with women who have not had a breast biopsy:

Lobular carcinoma in situ (LCIS), according to strict criteria, uncommon compared with ALH (see above)

Each of these histologic diagnoses has its own associations with clinical presentation, detectability, and precision of diagnosis. For example, sclerosing adenosis may be diagnosed with little histologic change, but the indication of increased risk demands specific criteria that have been linked to cancer risk after prolonged follow-up.

associated with a significant increase in risk, there is some evidence to suggest that recurrent large cysts in the immediate pre-menopausal period may be associated with a risk comparable to that of the atypical hyperplasias.

Also of special concern is sclerosing adenosis, as well-developed sclerosing adenosis is associated with an increased risk of breast cancer that is somewhat higher than that of the other elements associated with the fibrocystic complex. Sclerosing adenosis alone approaches a risk of two times, although this has not been confirmed in very many studies, and requires precise histopathologic confirmation of findings including enlarged lobular units and other features. These findings are reviewed in publications by Hartmann and colleagues and Fitzgibbons et al. Fitzgibbons and colleagues clearly discuss that these risk associations evolve with time, as some associations are found only in solitary studies, and are not confirmed in subsequent studies using different sets of patients.

Many studies have demonstrated the importance of hyperplasia without atypia as an indicator of slightly increased risk. This group may be more important than the smaller group of women with atypical hyperplasia. Approximately 25% of women who were biopsied in both the pre-and post-mammographic eras have hyperplasia without atypia, with atypical hyperplasia found in 4–5%.

The specifically defined hyperplasias, atypical lobular hyperplasia (ALH) and atypical ductal hyperplasia (ADH), are becoming recognized as having separate risk implications. ALH has a slightly greater risk of subsequent breast cancer than ADH, although the diagnosis of ALH in a woman after the age of 55 may have less significance. Figure 3.1 presents the information from a group of women followed by Dupont and Page in Nashville, Tennessee. The authors present the graph as restricted to women younger than age 55 because this particular cohort does not have a large number of women older than that. The information is and validated for the majority of the women in this group who are aged 40–55 years at the time of biopsy. Of note, in the NSABP P-1 (National Surgical Adjuvant Breast Project) trial evaluating

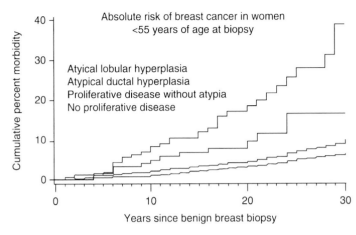

Figure 3.1. Cumulative risk of invasive breast cancer after benign breast biopsy. Cumulative morbidity of the development of invasive breast cancer with prolonged follow-up from the Nashville cohort for 2000 (preliminary data of extended follow-up courtesy of WD Dupont and DL Page). The analysis of maximal likelihood estimates gives risk ratios compared with women without proliferative disease of 4.4 for ALH (95% confidence interval 3.1–6.3), 2.9 for ADH (95% CI 1.9–4.5), and 1.4 for PDWA (95% CI 1.2–1.7). The P value for all of these values is less than 0/0.001 for the atypical hyperplasias and approximately 0.0003 for the larger group of women with proliferative disease without atypia. Note: The present restriction to women younger than 55 years of age at the time of biopsy is made in order to make very clear that the majority of women from this particular cohort were less than 55 at the time of biopsy, and that these numbers, at least with regard to ALH, are more important before the age of 55. There is good evidence that this risk of ALH falls after the age of 55. ALH: atypical lobular hyperplasia; ADH: atypical ductal hyperplasia; PDWA: proliferative disease without atypia (Data from Page et al., 1985).

breast cancer risk reduction with tamoxifen use, women who identified themselves as having had atypical lobular hyperplasia or lobular carcinoma in situ were found to have a greater reduction in cancer development than other women in the study. Lobular carcinoma in situ (LCIS) is a very uncommon diagnosis of very advanced changes, and there is evidence that the risk of cancer associated with LCIS is slightly higher than that shown for ALH in Fig. 3.1. Both LCIS and ALH are significant risk factors for the later development of breast cancer, which is certainly bilateral, but may slightly favor the breast in which the original biopsy identified the atypical hyperplasia.

Hormone Contraception

Results of pooled analyses of the many epidemiologic studies suggest that current and recent use of combined oral contraceptives minimally increases the risk of breast cancer as compared to women who have never used them. None of these relative risks were greater than 1.24, and there was general agreement that this excess risk declined after cessation of use and is no longer evident 10 years after the last use. Therefore, risk of oral contraceptive therapy is minimal. There is not reliable identification of a subset or differences with age association, and thus, oral contraceptive use remains a minimal risk factor after many studies.

Post-menopausal Hormone Therapy

Few areas of medicine have received as much attention as post-menopausal hormone therapy and its association with breast cancer risk. Major studies over the past several years, including the Women's Health Initiative (WHI), have demonstrated that especially combined estrogen/progestin hormone replacement therapy is associated with an increased risk of developing breast cancer, although the alteration in risk is small.

Unopposed hormone replacement therapy with estrogen alone to aid in prevention of osteoporosis and prevent menopausal symptoms gained widespread popularity in the United States through the 1970s. Concern with endometrial carcinomas has been balanced against the observations that risk of death, as opposed to presentation of low-stage endometrial carcinomas, appeared well balanced. Pooled analyses of many epidemiologic studies in the late 1990s demonstrated that estrogen replacement increased risk of breast cancer with increasing duration of use, that use for 5 years did not increase risk more than 50%, and use for up to 10 years might approach a doubling of risk. A consistent observation has been that carcinomas diagnosed in women who are current or recent users tended to be less advanced clinically and to be estrogen, receptor positive tumors of better prognosis than those diagnosed in non-users. A slightly greater increased risk has been observed when progestin is added, although whether this risk is more than double is uncertain, considering the shifting risk of comparison users of estrogen alone.

The Women's Health Initiative Study recruited healthy women and has reported on many women who essentially began the study in their late 50s, whereas younger women from these studies have yet to be reported. The estrogen-progestin arm of this study was abruptly ended in July 2002 with the finding of an estimated a 25% increased risk of breast carcinomas in that particular cohort. There has been a lack of understanding an estimated possibility of increased risk of more advanced cancers in these women. In fact, the comparison of users to the non-users of combined therapy did not show a meaningful difference with regard to size of carcinomas or lymph node involvement. When the estrogen-only arm was published, many were surprised that the risk of the users of estrogen was actually reduced compared to non-users. It is now accepted that combined hormone replacement therapy does increase breast cancer risk and the routine use of the combined agent is not recommended. However, estrogen alone has little risk unless prolonged over 5 years. Use of post-menopausal hormonal therapy has become a carefully weighted decision based on the individual woman's potential benefits and risks associated with hormone use, and one that requires ongoing evaluation.

Risk Assessment Models

Models for risk assessment are available to aid the clinician in identifying women at increased risk for breast cancer. Models are available to assess cancer risk based on personal and family history or family history alone, as well as to assess the likelihood of hereditary breast/ovarian cancer syndrome associated with mutations in *BRCA1* and *BRCA2*. All of the models, whether to identify those at increased risk of developing breast cancer or the risk of carrying a mutation in a cancer susceptibility gene, have significant limitations and represent an educated guess or likelihood for that individual woman. In reality, her risk will either be zero or one hundred percent.

Gail Model

The Gail Model, published in 1989, was created to aid in evaluating an individual woman's risk of developing breast cancer from a given age over a specified time interval. The model used personal risk factors, including current age, age at menarche, age at first live birth, number of previous breast biopsies, and number of first-degree relatives with breast cancer. The model was later adapted to include pathologic indicators of risk, atypical ductal hyperplasia, and lobular carcinoma in situ. Specific patient characteristics are entered into the model, and a probability is calculated for the risk of developing breast cancer in 5 year increments, along with the rate for a patient of the same age without specific risk factors. The model was developed from primarily white women who were being examined annually through the Breast Cancer Detection and Demonstration Project (BCDDP) in the United States. The model has been utilized in breast cancer prevention trials, the National Surgical Adjuvant Breast Project (NSAPB), and the Study of Tamoxifen and Raloxifene (STAR) trials in the United States. The adapted model (incorporating pathologic finding of atypical hyperplasia and race) is available at http://www.cancer.gov/bcrisktool.

Claus Model

The Claus Model is a useful tool in evaluating risks of breast cancer in women with a family history of breast or ovarian cancer. Claus et al. used the data from the CASH (Cancer and Steroid Hormone) Study by the Centers for Disease Control in the United States to predict the cumulative probability of developing breast cancer by age based on the age at diagnoses of breast cancer in relatives. The Claus model assumes autosomal dominant inheritance of highly-penetrant breast cancer susceptibility genes.

The Claus tables incorporate maternal and paternal family history, and include second-degree relatives and family history of ovarian cancer. In the absence of identification of an hereditary cancer syndrome with useful predictive testing, the Claus tables can serve as a guide to estimate breast cancer risk.

BRCAPRO

The identification of genes associated with hereditary susceptibility to breast and ovarian cancer has allowed for clarification of risk in some families. Clinical testing for *BRCA1* and *BRCA2* mutations has been available since the mid-1990s. BRCAPRO is a model that utilizes Bayesian analysis and previously published models to predict the likelihood of finding a mutation in *BRCA1* or *BRCA2*, as well as the risks of breast and ovarian cancer based on family history. A user-friendly version of the model called CaGene is available for download at http://astor.som.jhmi.edu/BayesMendel/brcapro.html through David Euhus at University of Texas Southwestern. This model incorporates age at diagnosis of breast and ovarian cancer in the family, bilaterality of breast cancer, and Ashkenazi Jewish heritage in evaluating risk.

Frank/Myriad Model

The Frank Model uses data from over 10,000 samples tested through Myriad Genetics, Inc. in estimating the likelihood of identifying a deleterious mutation in *BRCA1* or *BRCA2*. This model is updated by the company and is available on the website at http://www.myriadtests.com/provider/brcamutation-prevalence.htm

It provides a quick risk estimate, and includes breast and ovarian cancer in the family, separated by age at diagnosis of breast cancer at younger than age 50 or greater.

Breast Cancer Risk Assessment and Consultation

Cancer risk assessment is a process of gathering information from the patient's personal and family history, and evaluating his or her risk based on information from the available literature, utilizing appropriate risk assessment models, and providing information to aid in making decisions for risk reduction or surveillance, in hopes of preventing cancers or identifying cancers earlier. Genetic testing is an option for many to clarify risk and provide valuable information for the family. As this is such a time-consuming process, in most settings this service is provided by advanced practice nurses with special interest and training in cancer genetics, or by genetic counselors with special interest and training in cancer. The service is often provided in consultation with other medical specialists.

The process for cancer risk assessment involves initial information gathering. The patient is asked to gather their family history with emphasis on cancer diagnoses, age at diagnoses, age and cause of death, or other surgeries or procedures that might alter risk (such as oophorectomy). The family history is then reviewed and documented in pedigree form. In addition, the patient's personal medical history is reviewed and cancer diagnoses are documented with pathology reports or pathology review when possible. Menstrual and hormonal histories are also reviewed. Finally, the patient's expectations of the consultation are discussed, as well as what can reasonably be accomplished. It is important to recognize the patient's personal experiences of cancer in her family or other individuals in her life.

The educational component of the process is varied based on the individual's needs at the time, but may include a review of cancer risk factors in general. This includes breast and ovarian cancer, and the lifetime and age-adjusted risks of cancer in the general population, so that they can be seen in the context of the risk to the individual. A brief discussion may include types of risk that may be used to express risk of cancer and the models used to evaluate that risk. The limitations of the models in individual assessment is also addressed. Recommendations for cancer screening or options available to decrease risk are reviewed with the patient, including the possible limitations of current screening or risk-reducing measures.

Information about the hereditary cancer syndromes under consideration is reviewed. If the family history is suggestive of hereditary breast/ovarian cancer syndrome associated with *BRCA1* and *BRCA2*, then facilitation of genetic testing for mutations in these genes is offered. The likelihood of identifying a mutation in *BRCA1* or *BRCA2* according to the available models is reviewed. Testing may be considered despite the risk of testing positive being small according to the models. Limitations of the models may be evident in families where there are few relatives, few female relatives, or limited information about the family. Consideration of families or individuals to test is not always a straightforward process. Individuals of Ashkenazi Jewish heritage have an increased likelihood of carrying one of three founder mutations in *BRCA1* and *BRCA2*, and testing for these three mutations in this group will identify 95% of those with a mutation. Table 3.5 lists characteristics of families appropriate for consideration of genetic testing. The decision is likely to be very personal for the patient and family members. The costs, process, timing, and limitations of testing are reviewed. Testing usually involves complete gene sequencing for *BRCA1* and *BRCA2* and evaluation for genomic rearrangements not seen on sequencing. Testing is expensive, and it takes several weeks for results to be available. The test results can be positive for a deleterious mutation, or may identify variants of uncertain clinical significance or no mutation at all. It is important for the patient to understand this prior to testing. Ideally, an affected family member is tested initially, and if a deleterious mutation is identified, then unaffected family members can be tested with definitive results. A negative test only has

TABLE 3.5. Characteristics of families and individuals appropriate for consideration of genetic testing for *BRCA1* and *BRCA2* mutations.

Family history with multiple cases of breast and/or ovarian cancer
Family or personal history of bilateral breast cancer
Family or personal history of individual with both breast and ovarian cancer
Family or personal history of male breast cancer
Family history of more than one person with ovarian cancer
Multiple affected family members, autosomal dominant pattern of inheritance on pedigree
Family or personal history of breast and/or ovarian cancer and Ashkenazi Jewish heritage
Family or personal history of cancers diagnosed at younger than expected ages

significant meaning in the setting of a previously identified mutation in the family.

The prevalence of clinically significant *BRCA1* and *BRCA2* mutations varies with populations. In the United States, this may be around 1/500. In individuals of Ashkenazi Jewish heritage, this is 1/40. Women identified with mutations in *BRCA1* and *BRCA2* have significantly increased risks of breast and ovarian cancers. The risks associated with mutations in these genes are still being characterized. These are reviewed in Table 3.6. Some families have cancer pedigrees consistent with hereditary breast/ ovarian cancer syndrome, but test negative for mutations in *BRCA1* and *BRCA2* with clinically available tests. A recent study demonstrated that for very high-risk families (i.e. those with four cases of breast or ovarian cancer, with negative commercial testing for *BRCA1* and *BRCA2* when screened for genomic rearrangements in *BRCA1* and *BRCA2*, as well as mutations in *CHEK2*, *TP53*, and *PTEN*) 17%, were found to have previously undetected mutations. Of these, 12% were previously undetected genomic rearrangements in *BRCA1* or *BRCA2*, 5% had *CHEK2*

TABLE 3.6. Selected risks of cancer associated with BRCA1 and BRCA2 mutations (%) (Easton et al., 1995, 1999; Ford). Breast cancer by age (women)

	BRCA1	BRCA2	AJ (not selected for FH)		General Population (US)[a]		
			BRCA1	BRCA2	BRCA2[a]	BRCA1 or BRCA1	BRCA2[b]
30			3		–	–	–
40	19	12	21		17		
50	50	28	39		34	33	2
60	64	48	58		48		
70	85	84	69		74	56	7
Risk of contralateral breast cancer					Women who have had breast cancer (not BRCA1/BRCA2)		
5 Years after diagnosis	20	12					2.5–5
By age 70	60	52					
Risk of breast cancer in men		6–10					0.05
Risk of ovarian cancer							
40	0.6	–	3		2		
50	22	0.4	21		2		
60	30	7.4	40		0.6		

(continued)

TABLE 3.6. (continued)

Breast cancer by age (women)

| | BRCA1 | BRCA2 | AJ (not selected for FH) | | General Population (US)[a] | | |
			BRCA1	BRCA2[a]	BRCA1 or BRCA2	BRCA2[b]
70	63	27	46	12		
80			54	23		<2
Prostate cancer						
70		7.5			16	
80		19.8			39	~8

Other cancers increased with *BRCA*: gallbladder, bile duct, stomach, melanoma, buccal cavity, pharynx, pancreatic
[a]King et al. (2003).
[b]Struewing et al. (1997).

mutations, and 1% had *TP53* mutations. Mutations in the *CHEK2* gene are associated with increased risk of breast cancer. Testing for mutations in this gene are now clinically available, although the cancer risks associated with such mutations are still being characterized.

Breast cancer is a component of other hereditary cancer syndromes in addition to hereditary breast/ovarian syndrome associated with *BRCA1* and *BRCA2*. Care must be taken in cancer risk assessment/counseling and pedigree interpretation to consider other hereditary cancer syndromes. Cowden's syndrome is an under-recognized syndrome associated with an increased risk of breast and thyroid cancers, and mutations in the *PTEN* gene. Li-Fraumeni is a syndrome associated with multiple cancers, many of which can occur in childhood, that are related to mutations in TP53 gene. The cancers associated with this syndrome include adrenocortical carcinoma, sarcomas, breast cancer, brain cancer, and leukemias. Another syndrome associated with hamartomatous polyps and increased risk of breast cancer is Peutz-Jeghers syndrome, which is related to mutations in *STK11/LKB1*. Although these syndromes are more rare, one must take care to recognize the possibility of other syndromes and offer appropriate testing and surveillance for the potential consequences of such syndromes.

Recommendations for Screening Women at Increased Risk

It is now well established that there is benefit to screening women for breast cancer, including clinical breast examination and mammographic screening. By definition, general population screening recommendations are for women without known risk factors or for those with specific breast problems, but should be encouraged for all women.

Women identified with clinically significant increased risk should be offered more intensive screening with mammography offered at an earlier age. In specific circumstances,

MRI of the breast may be offered in addition to mammographic screening. Instruction and encouragement of breast self-examination may be offered. Clinical breast examination may be offered every 6 months rather than annually, or even more often in women who are uncomfortable or too anxious to do monthly self-examinations. The utility of screening and ideal management of women at very high risk of developing breast cancer, such as those at risk due to hereditary susceptibility, is an ongoing endeavor. Recommendations include monthly breast self-examination, annual or semi-annual clinical breast examinations, and mammography beginning at ages 25–35 or based on the family history. In addition, prompt evaluation of any abnormal findings is appropriate in women of increased risk. For syndromes associated with increased risks of other cancers, surveillance or risk-reducing measures should be appropriate to cancer risks.

Interventions for Decreasing the Risk of Breast Cancer

Ideally, individuals at very high risk of breast cancer are managed in clinical settings that are experienced in caring for such patients. Increased surveillance for breast cancer is aimed at identifying cancers earlier. Measures to decrease risk may also be an option. Medications such as tamoxifen or raloxifene may be considered. These medications are associated with significant side effects, and one must carefully balance the risks and potential benefits for the individual woman. Risk-reducing mastectomy is another option for women at very high risk. This is an extreme measure, one that should not be taken without careful consideration and repeated consultation. A significant part of this decision for many women is their personal experience with cancer. It should also be noted that oophorectomy has been associated with a decreased risk of breast cancer in very high-risk women with hereditary breast/ ovarian cancer syndrome.

Conclusion

We have many tools available to help in identifying women at significantly increased risk of developing breast cancer. Identification and careful assessment of an individual woman's risks can provide the opportunity to alleviate anxiety and distress, and offer increased surveillance and measures to decrease risk.

Selected Readings

American Cancer Society (2000) Cancer Facts and Figures. American Cancer Society, Atlanta, GA

Berry DA, Parmigiani G, Sanchez J, et al. (1997) Probability of carrying a mutation of breast-ovarian cancer gene BRCA1 based on family history. J Natl Cancer Inst 89:227–238

Claus EB, Risch N, Thompson WD (1994) Autosomal dominant inheritance of early-onset breast cancer: implications for risk prediction. Cancer 73:643–651

Collaborative Group on Hormonal Factors in Breast Cancer (1996) Breast cancer and hormonal contraceptives: collaborative reanalysis of individual data on 53, 297 women with breast cancer and 100,239 women without breast cancer from 54 epidemiologic studies. Lancet 347:1713–1727

Dupont WD (1989) Converting relative risks to absolute risks: a graphical approach. Stat Med 8:641–651

Dupont WD, Plummer WD (1996) Understanding the relationship between relative and absolute risk. Cancer 77:2193–2199

Easton DF, Ford D, Bishop T, and the Breast Cancer Linkage Consortium (1995) Breast and ovarian cancer incidence in BRCA1-mutation carriers. Am J Hum Genet 56:265–271

Easton D et al., and the Breast Cancer Linkage Consortium (1999) Cancer risks in BRCA2 mutation carriers. J Natl Cancer Inst 91:1310–1316

Feuer EJ, Wun LM, Boring CC, et al. (1993) The lifetime risk of developing breast cancer. J Natl Cancer Inst 85:892

Fitzgibbons PL, Henson DE, Hutter RV (1998) Benign breast changes and the risk for subsequent breast cancer: an update of the 1985 consensus statement. Cancer Committee of the College of American Pathologists. Arch Pathol Lab Med 122:1053–1055

Ford D, Easton DF, Bishop T, Narod SA, Goldgar DE, and the Breast Cancer Linkage Consortium (1994) Risk of breast cancer in BRCA1 mutation carriers. Lancet 343:692–695

Ford D, Easton DF, Stratton M, et al. (1998) Genetic heterogeneity and penetrance analysis of the BRCA1 and BRCA2 genes in breast cancer families. Am J Hum Genet 62:676–689

Frank TS, Deffenbaugh AM, Reid JE, et al. (2002) Clinical characteristics of individuals with germline mutations in BRCA1 and BRCA2: analysis of 10,000 individuals. J Clin Oncol 20:1480–1490

Gail MH, Brinton LA, Byar DP, et al. (1989) Projecting individualized probabilities of developing breast cancer for white females who are being examined annually. J Nat Cancer Inst 81:1879–1886

Hartmann LC, Sellers TA, Frost MH, et al. (2005) Benign breast disease and the risk of breast cancer. N Engl J Med 353:229–237

Henderson IC (1993) Risk factors for cancer development. Cancer 71(7):2127–2140

King M-C, Marks JH, Mandell JB, for the New York Breast Cancer Study Group (2003) Breast and ovarian cancer risks due to inherited mutations in BRCA1 and BRCA2. Science 302:643–646

McLaren BK, Schuyler PA, Sanders ME, et al. (2006) Excellent survival, cancer type, and Nottingham grade after atypical lobular hyperplasia on initial breast biopsy. Cancer 107:1227–1233

Page DL, Dupont WD, Rogers LW, Rados MS (1985) Atypical hyperplastic lesions of the female breast. Cancer 55:2698–2708

Page DL, Schuyler PA, Dupont WD, et al. (2003) Atypical lobular hyperplasia as a unilateral predictor of breast cancer risk: a retrospective cohort study. Lancet 361:125–129

Reis LAG, Kosary CL, Hankey BF, et al. (eds) (1998) SEER Cancer Statistics Review. (1973–1975). National Cancer Institute, Bethesda, MD, Table IV-9

Reis LAG, Miller BA, Hankey BF, Kosary CL, Harras A, Edwards BK (1999) SEER Cancer Statistics Review (1973–1996). National Cancer Institute, Bethesda, MD, Table IV-2

Struewing JP, Hartge P, Wacholder W, et al. (1997) The risk of cancer associated with specific mutations in BRCA1 and BRCA2 among Ashkenazi Jews. New Engl J Med 336:1401–1408

Walsh T, Casadei S, Coats KH (2006) Spectrum of mutations in *BRCA1*, *BRCA2*, *CHEK2*, and *TP53* in families at high risk of breast cancer. JAMA 295:1379–1388

Writing Group for the Women's Health Initiative Investigation (2002) Risks and benefits of estrogen plus progestin in healthy postmenopausal women. Principal results from the women's health initiative randomized controlled trial. JAMA 288:321–333

4
Carcinoma In Situ of the Breast: Ductal and Lobular Origin

Theresa A. Graves and Kirby I. Bland

Pearls and Pitfalls

Lobular Carcinoma In Situ (LCIS)

- LCIS represents a 1% per year lifetime risk factor for the development of bilateral breast cancer.
- LCIS is a potential precursor to invasive breast carcinoma in unusual circumstances (pleomorphic LCIS).
- Observation with lifelong clinical and radiographic follow-up represents the consensus for treatment.
- Bilateral prophylactic mastectomy is an operative alternative; hereditary factors may influence this choice. There is no role for unilateral mastectomy in LCIS.
- Chemoprevention with tamoxifen or raloxifene may reduce the incidence of subsequent carcinoma by 50% or more.
- Radiation therapy and axillary dissection play no therapeutic or diagnostic role in patients with LCIS.

Ductal Carcinoma In Situ (DCIS)

- The majority of DCIS lesions are detected mammographically as clustered microcalcifications; however, the volume of microcalcifications may underestimate the extent of disease.

K.I. Bland et al. (eds.), *Surgery in Breast Cancer and Melanoma*, DOI 10.1007/978-1-84996-435-7_4, © Springer-Verlag London Limited 2011

- Stereotactic core needle biopsy (CNB) is the preferred diagnostic procedure for nonpalpable mammographic abnormalities.
- Total mastectomy (TM) is considered curative, with a subsequent disease-specific mortality of 0–1%.
- Breast-conserving surgery (BCS) is an alternative for localized DCIS.
- Complete resection should be ensured radiographically and pathologically.
- The addition of adjuvant radiation therapy to BCS is based on prognostic factors that influence local recurrence (LR).
- Excision alone may be appropriate for selected women with small, low-grade lesions and adequate surgical margins (consider clinical trial).
- Axillary dissection is not indicated in DCIS; however, in large high-grade DCIS lesions requiring mastectomy, sentinel lymph node biopsy (SLNB) may avoid reoperation if invasion is identified.
- Approximately 50% of all LRs present as invasive cancer with a 10-year disease-specific mortality up to 15% for the invasive cancer.
- Tamoxifen may be considered a risk-reduction treatment for both ipsilateral recurrence and contralateral breast cancer.

Introduction: Lobular Carcinoma In Situ

LCIS is a clinically occult noninvasive breast lesion arising from the lobules and terminal ducts of the breast. While the true incidence of LCIS is unknown due to a lack of clinical and radiographic signs, a 2.6-to 4-fold increase in the frequency of LCIS has been attributed to the increased use of screening mammography, as well as a greater recognition of this pathologic entity. With a greater understanding of the natural history of this disease, clinicians now recognize LCIS as a risk factor for the development of breast carcinoma rather than a precursor lesion. Consequently, a nonoperative approach was adopted with lifelong surveillance as the consensus for treatment. Bilateral mastectomy continues to be offered to patients as an opportunity for surgical prevention; however, this represents overtreatment, as the majority of women do not develop a subsequent malignancy.

The results of the NSABP P-1 and P-2 trials have demonstrated a significant reduction in breast cancer incidence with the use of the estrogen receptor modulators (tamoxifen and raloxifene) in high-risk patients, including those with LCIS. This has allowed an effective alternative to observation or bilateral mastectomy.

Natural History

Relevant to the management of LCIS is the risk for subsequent development of an invasive cancer resulting in cancer-specific mortality. The relative risk for the development of invasive breast carcinoma over the baseline index population has been estimated at 3- to 4.2-fold. LCIS has a 23–30% risk for subsequent cancer at 15–20 years following diagnosis, whereas DCIS has a 30–50% chance for subsequent cancer at 10–15 years, highlighting the variance in the lead-time bias of the two lesions. Moreover, there appears to be a greater frequency of contralateral disease with LCIS, and subsequent malignancies may be either lobular or ductal. Based on a recent analysis of Surveillance, Epidemiology, and End Results (SEER) data, a proportionately greater incidence of invasive lobular carcinoma (23.1%) is diagnosed in patients with LCIS compared to that seen in the general population (6.5%). Infiltrating ductal carcinoma still represents the majority (49.7%) of subsequent breast cancers identified following an LCIS diagnosis. The occurrence of infiltrating ductal cancer and the bilateral equality of risk, combined with the observation that the majority of LCIS patients do not develop invasive breast cancer, support the hypothesis that LCIS represents a risk factor rather than a precursor of breast cancer.

Treatment

Until recently, surgical excision for LCIS diagnosed by CNB was questioned. Increasing evidence for a significant rate of upgrade in the diagnosis of DCIS or invasive cancer following an excision for LCIS and atypical lobular hyperplasia, similar to that of atypical ductal hyperplasia (ADH), has prompted the recommendation for surgical excision for each of these lesions. Clearance of surgical margins with re-excision is not clinically relevant as the multifocal and bilateral nature of LCIS has been documented.

Assuming that LCIS represents a risk factor for the development of breast carcinoma, careful observation with lifelong surveillance is the current standard treatment. The observation that women with LCIS are 5.3 times more likely to develop invasive lobular carcinoma and 0.8 times less likely to develop infiltrating ductal carcinoma compared to women with DCIS, however, may raise some doubts regarding a precursor status. At a minimum, surveillance for LCIS includes annual mammography, clinical breast examination at 6- to 12-month intervals, breast self-examination, and diagnostic evaluation as necessary. Breast magnetic resonance imaging (MRI) has shown promise in genetically high-risk patients in identifying clinically and mammographically occult lesions, but has a similar rate of false-positive findings to mammography.

Bilateral prophylactic mastectomy with or without immediate reconstruction remains an option for a subset of patients with LCIS. High-risk candidates include those with an additional risk of family history or *BRCA1/BRCA2* genetic abnormality carriers. Patients unwilling or unable to accept the lifelong 1% per year risk of a subsequent cancer or maintain adequate surveillance may also choose this surgical option. Partial mastectomy with radiation currently has no therapeutic role. Further, axillary dissection is unwarranted, as nodal metastases occur in less than 1% of patients.

Data from the NSABP P-01 prevention trial included 826 patients with LCIS, with a median follow-up of 55 months. A 56% reduction in the incidence of invasive breast cancer was noted among women taking tamoxifen compared with those receiving placebo. Raloxifene was found to be as effective as tamoxifen in the NSABP P-02 (STAR) trial for reduction of invasive breast cancer; however, there was a statistically non-significant higher risk of noninvasive breast cancer in patients receiving raloxifene. Diminished risks of thromboembolic events and cataracts, and a statistically non-significant trend for decreased incidence of uterine cancer, was noted in the raloxifene group. These chemoprevention strategies offer therapeutic alternatives that bridge the management extremes of observation and bilateral mastectomy. NSABP P-04 trial will randomize high-risk, postmenopausal women, including patients with LCIS, to receive either raloxifene or an aromatase inhibitor as a chemopreventative agent.

Recommendation from the National Comprehensive Cancer Network (NCCN) clinical practice guidelines for LCIS are outlined in Fig. 4.1.

Outcome

Data from observational studies indicate a lifetime cancer-specific mortality as great as 7% associated, with observation alone, with a 1% per year risk for developing an invasive cancer. However, a more recent long-term study has indicated a substantially lower (1%) mortality risk. With the use of chemopreventive agents, this mortality risk may be further reduced. Bilateral prophylactic mastectomy confers an approximately 90% reduction in the development of subsequent breast carcinoma with negligible cancer-specific mortality, but will overtreat the majority of women who would never progress to an invasive cancer.

Introduction: Ductal Carcinoma In Situ

DCIS of the breast represents a proliferation of malignant cells of the ducts and terminal lobular units of the breast that have not transgressed the ductal basement membrane.

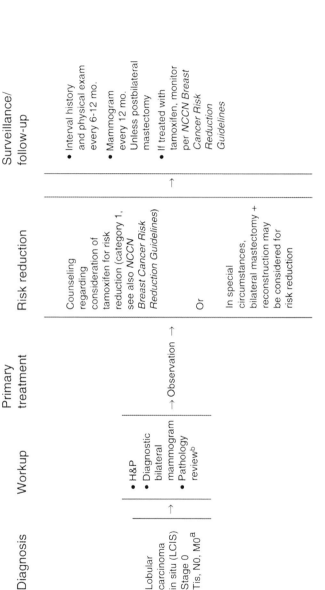

Diagnosis	Workup	Primary treatment	Risk reduction	Surveillance/follow-up
Lobular carcinoma in situ (LCIS) Stage 0 Tis, N0, M0[a]	• H&P • Diagnostic bilateral mammogram • Pathology review[b]	→ Observation →	Counseling regarding consideration of tamoxifen for risk reduction (category 1, see also *NCCN Breast Cancer Risk Reduction Guidelines*) Or In special circumstances, bilateral mastectomy + reconstruction may be considered for risk reduction	→	• Interval history and physical exam every 6-12 mo. • Mammogram every 12 mo. Unless postbilateral mastectomy • If treated with tamoxifen, monitor per *NCCN Breast Cancer Risk Reduction Guidelines*

FIGURE 4.1. Recommendations from the NCCN Breast Cancer Clinical Practice Guideline (For the most current version, go to www.nccn.org) (Reproduced from Anderson et al., 2006. With permission from the NCCN (2.2006) Breast Cancer Clinical Practice Guidelines in Oncology. 2006 National Comprehensive Cancer Network, Inc. To view the most recent and complete version of the guideline, go online to www.nccn.org).

The widespread availability of high-resolution screening mammography has increased the diagnosis of DCIS by tenfold in the past 2 decades and accounts for approximately 20% of all mammographically detected breast malignancies. As mammographic screening has become a national health priority, this trend is expected to continue.

Historically, this poorly understood breast cancer was predominantly treated with mastectomy. The increase in breast-conserving therapy (BCT) for invasive cancer has spurred a movement toward a similar management for DCIS; however, limited data exists about the natural history of DCIS to use as a basis for treatment decisions. DCIS is the most rapidly enlarging cohort of breast cancer with more than 56,000 new cases diagnosed in the USA in 2003. The majority of these new cases are nonpalpable and discovered mammographically. As an in situ disease, DCIS does not express the full malignant phenotype, lacking invasion and metastatic potential. Mastectomy is considered curative, with a 0–1% disease-specific mortality. However, an invasive LR following BCT carries the risk of increased breast cancer mortality.

Clinical Presentation

Previously, DCIS presented with a palpable mass, bloody or serous nipple discharge, or Paget's disease. With high-resolution mammography, nearly 90% of DCIS is detected as clinically occult lesions with clustered microcalcifications (76%), soft tissue densities (11%), or both (13%). While mammography is an excellent diagnostic tool, its specificity in distinguishing benign from malignant lesions is only 50–60% and may frequently underestimate the extent of disease. These microcalcifications tend to represent the comedo necrosis evident in grade III lesions. Indeterminant or pleomorphic calcifications may also represent DCIS. Microcalcifications may also represent benign fibrocystic changes, such as sclerosing adenosis, with DCIS identified only incidentally and not associated with the microcalcifications. Consequently, it is critical that the biopsy specimen, whether open or core, undergo specimen radiography, and that the pathologists verify whether the DCIS is associated with the microcalcifications.

Preoperative Evaluation

Diagnosis

Image-directed procedures are needed for both diagnosis and treatment. Stereotactic CNBs of the breast are the recommended initial step in diagnosing nonpalpable mammographic abnormalities. Not all lesions are amenable to stereotactic biopsy, owing to the technical limitations of low-volume breasts or very superficial or deep lesions. When stereotactic biopsy is employed, multiple cores (9–11 gauge, optimally with vacuum assistance) should be obtained to ensure adequate sampling of the micro-calcifications. If all microcalcifications are removed, a wire clip should be left as a marker for future localization and excision. Complete surgical excision of these lesions often results in upstaging of ADH to carcinoma (both DCIS and infiltrating ductal carcinoma) in 10–50% of cases and of DCIS to an invasive carcinoma in 10–15% of cases. When stereotactic biopsy is not possible or returns a pathologic diagnosis of ADH or DCIS, a wire localization open biopsy is necessary. This will allow a precise diagnosis and may achieve therapeutic breast conservation for the patient with DCIS only.

Pathology

The classification of DCIS histopathologically has slowly evolved; traditionally, it has been based on an architectural pattern with two main categories: comedo and noncomedo (cribriform, micropapillary, papillary, and solid). Comedo lesions exhibit prominent necrosis and tumor cells with pleomorphic nuclei and higher mitotic rates. Noncomedo types typically are of low nuclear grade without prominent necrosis. Comedo lesions more frequently have microinvasion, a greater degree of angiogenesis, and higher proliferative rate. Recently, pathologists have proposed new classifications based on nuclear grade and the presence or absence of necrosis, which may better delineate prognostic factors to guide optimal therapy.

Breast Imaging

Standard mammographic views often underestimate the volume of disease, and magnification views are critical in the evaluation of microcalcifications. Multifocality (foci in proximity to the index lesion) may be treated with breast conservation, whereas multicentric lesions (foci located in a separate quadrant) have a negative impact on the success of breast conservation. Holland has reported that the majority of lesions demonstrate multifocal, and not multicentric, patterns. The well-differentiated DCIS lesion is more likely to demonstrate a multifocal pattern than the poorly differentiated tumor (70% vs. 10%). MRI with contrast enhancement has shown promise in better defining the extent and distribution of DCIS in the breast. MRI may be particularly useful in evaluating for multicentricity, residual disease, or occult invasion, thereby assisting in surgical management.

Surgical Options

Surgical therapy for DCIS is based upon breast imaging, patient factors, and the histopathologic sampling generally provided by image-guided biopsy. Surgical options include mastectomy with or without immediate reconstruction, or excision with negative margins to be followed by observation (rarely) or adjuvant breast radiation. Mastectomy (total-simple) remains the most aggressive surgical therapy for DCIS and the standard by which the outcomes of all other therapies are measured. Indications for mastectomy include: multicentric disease with two or more foci, diffuse malignant-appearing (or proven) microcalcifications, and cases with persistently positive margins after surgical re-excision. Patient factors that preclude the use of radiation therapy constitute a relative indication for mastectomy and include a history of collagen vascular disease, previous irradiation to the breast or chest, and pregnancy. Mastectomy provides maximal risk reduction of LR but may represent surgical overtreatment for the majority of patients with small mammographically detected lesions.

Indications for BCS include DCIS detected mammo-graphically or a localized palpable lesion without multi-centricity or diffuse microcalcifications. The decision for the addition of radiation to BCT is also based on the prognostic factors that influence LR and may be affected by radiation therapy.

A critical factor in preoperative management includes assessment of the patient's needs and expectations regarding breast preservation. Treatment should be tailored to patient preference and to an understanding that risk management is limited to local control. While BCT allows for a better cos-metic outcome compared with mastectomy, patients must be willing to accept the higher risk of LR associated with BCT. Approximately 50% of LR after BCT for DCIS presents as invasive carcinoma and may result in lower survival for patients treated initially with BCT.

Intraoperative Management

Mastectomy

TM may be performed with or without immediate recon-struction. The most significant recent advance in breast reconstruction has been the use of skin-sparing mastectomy, in which a TM, inclusive of the nipple and areola complex, is performed via a periareolar incision. Large retrospective studies have shown no increase in the local breast cancer recurrence rates. Although skin and nipple areolar complex-sparing procedures are being evaluated for DCIS, only limited LR data (approximately 3–5%) are available at this time. Axillary dissection is not necessary for the management of most patients with DCIS, as the incidence of nodal metastasis in pure DCIS is only 0–1%. The use of SLNB remains controversial and should be considered in the context of clinical trials. Clinically suspicious nodes and surgically removed sentinel lymph nodes should undergo touch-prep or frozen section, and the identification of a positive lymph node should prompt the completion of a level I/II lymph node dissection at the time of the original surgery. This approach is particularly advantageous when immediate reconstruction is planned.

Breast-Conserving Therapy

Crucial to BCT outcomes is excision with careful attention to margin status of the lesion, while maintaining acceptable cosmesis. Nonpalpable, mammographically detected lesions are excised following presurgical localization of the abnormality with a guide wire placed with the assistance of breast imaging. Accurate excision may be enhanced with multiple wire-bracketing of larger abnormalities. The exact location of the wire tip is assessed by triangulation using the post-wire, two-view mammograms. A curvilinear skin incision is made closest to the wire tip, and extensive tunneling should be avoided. The specimen is preferably removed in one piece, with precise anatomic orientation through clips, ties, or a six-color margin-inking scheme. Such marking is critical for correct marginal analysis and will greatly facilitate subsequent re-excision. Additional shave margins have been advocated to avoid false-positive margins identified in inking systems and to diminish re-excision rates. Intraoperative touch-preps are advocated by some as a measure to avoid re-excision for positive margins. The rate of re-excision for a positive or close (<1 mm) margin is estimated to be as high as 55%, and re-excision generally detracts from the overall cosmetic result. Re-approximation of the biopsy cavity and the utilization of more advanced oncoplastic techniques afford a better cosmetic outcome.

Intraoperative radiogram of the specimen should be obtained and correlated by the surgeon with the mammographer using perioperative imaging studies. While specimen radiography is not adequate for determining the pathological completeness of excision, two views in magnification enhance image resolution and may assist identification of microcalcifications (or mass) extending to the margins of the specimen. Thereafter, resection may be accomplished. The specimen radiograph should accompany the specimen to pathology to assist in accurately sampling the abnormality. Frozen-section examination of image-guided excision specimens is discouraged, as ADH or DCIS may be indistinguishable on frozen section and small foci of microinvasion may be missed. Metallic clips should be placed in the operating site to assist with precise localization of the tumor bed for adjuvant radiation therapy to the breast.

Preoperative Management

Technical Considerations

Simple (total) mastectomy patients who do not elect immediate reconstruction are managed with a single closed suction drain, which is removed when the volume of output diminishes to less than 30 ml/day. BCT rarely requires drainage. Management following immediate reconstruction is based on the form of reconstruction with tissue-transfer techniques requiring closer monitoring for viability of the transferred tissue.

Assessment of Risk Factors for Local Recurrence

The recurrence rate following mastectomy is 0–2%, whereas for BCT the reported rates range from 10% to 40%. Critical to the optimal management of patients pursuing BCT is minimizing the risk of local relapse. Events leading to local relapse are multifactorial, with technical, tumor-related, and patient-related factors playing roles in LR following BCT.

Resection Margins

The principal technical consideration for local control is achieving an adequate resection margin, which represents the distance between the DCIS tumor and the edge of the excised specimen. Postoperative mammogram and margin status are complementary in assessing the completeness of excision. As DCIS lacks invasive and metastatic potential, complete excision should produce a cure. Standardized methods of assessing histologic margins did not exist until the late 1980s and consequently, earlier studies failed to demonstrate margin status as a significant factor in local control. Silverstein reported a retrospective analysis of the influence of margin width on LR in DCIS from a prospective database. Patients were stratified by margin width (>10 mm, 1–9 mm, and <1 mm). In patients with margins greater than 10 mm, the addition of irradiation did not lower the recurrence rate, with an estimated 4% probability of recurrence at 8 years. The statistical power to detect a difference in this group, however, is low. In the 1–9 mm group, a 20% LR rate was noted at 8 years without adjuvant radiation and 12% with radiation (P = NS). In addition, the irradiated lesions were significantly larger and more likely to have comedo necrosis and were followed for 20 months longer than the nonirradiated group. Subsequent prospective studies from this favorable prognostic group have failed to validate the low risk of recurrence in patients treated *without* radiation.

DCIS resected with margins less than 1 mm resulted in a statistically significant decrease in recurrence from 58% to 30% with the addition of radiation. This is clinically irrelevant, however, as both rates are prohibitively high for BCT. Work by Holland and colleagues demonstrated that DCIS may have gaps or skip lesions measuring up to 10 mm or more, which also raises the question of adequacy of 1–2 mm margins. Patients are currently being enrolled in prospective protocols (RTOG trial 98-04 and ECOG trial E-5194) evaluating the use of excision alone in selected patients.

Tumor-Related Factors

Evidence of necrosis on histologic evaluation of DCIS has long been associated with poor prognosis and higher recurrence rates. It has recently been determined that cellular architecture and nuclear grade influence LR more predictably than does comedo-necrosis alone. Recurrences in high-grade groups occurred within a much shorter interval than those in the low-grade or intermediate groups. Solin reported a 5-year recurrence rate of 12% versus 3% for high-grade compared to low-grade lesions, respectively, but by 10 years the recurrence rates were not statistically different at 18% and 15%, supporting a difference in time to progression rather than potential to recur. Tumor size, like margin width, reflects the distribution of the disease and the ability of the surgeon to adequately excise the DCIS.

University of Southern California/Van Nuys Prognostic Index (USC/VNPI)

Silverstein incorporated the prognostic factors of nuclear grade and comedo-necrosis with tumor size and margin width to develop the USC/VNPI. This index identifies subgroups of patients who do not require radiation if BCT is chosen. Table 4.1 depicts the USC/VNPI scoring system with the total of three scores from each of the predictors ranging from a low of 4 to a high of 12. The scores are correlated with treatment recommendations based on the outcome of 706 DCIS patients treated with breast preservation. When patients were segregated by score into three groups (4, 5, or 6; 7, 8, or 9; 10, 11, or 12), the probability of LR was significantly different for each subgroup (Fig. 4.2). The patients with the lowest

TABLE 4.1. The USC/Van Nuys Prognostic Index scoring system. One to three points are awarded for each of four different predictors of local breast recurrence (size, margin width, pathologic classification, and age). Scores for each of the predictors are totaled to yield a VNPI score ranging from a low of 4 to a high of 12 (From Silverstein, 2003, Table 1).

Score	1	2	3
Size (mm)	≤15	16–40	≥41
Margin width(mm)	≥10	1–9	<1
Pathologic classification	Non-high grade without necrosis (nuclear grades 1 or 2)	Non-high grade with necrosis (nuclear grades 1 or 2)	High grade with or without necrosis (nuclear grade 3)
Age (year)	>60	40–60	<40

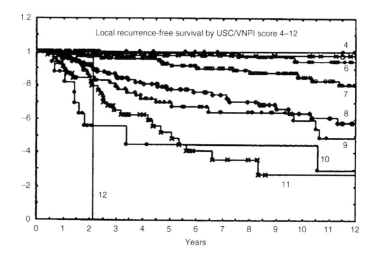

FIGURE 4.2. Probability of local recurrence-free survival for 706 breast conservation patients by modified USC/Van Nuys prognostic index score 4 to 12 (From Silverstein, 2003, Fig. 6).

scores had no difference in recurrence-free survival, regardless of the use of radiation, and could be considered for excision alone. The intermediate group demonstrated a statistically significant reduction ($P < 0.02$) in recurrence with radiation therapy. An unacceptably high rate of recurrence was seen in the highest subgroup when the patients were treated with BCT, and these patients should be considered for mastectomy.

Patient Factors

A 37% recurrence rate for women with a positive family history has been shown versus 9% for those without a family history of breast carcinoma. Younger women appear to have more aggressive tumor biology, as well as longer periods during which they are at risk for recurrence. The impact of youth and family history on recurrence risk is controversial and will require further evaluation and possible prospective analysis.

Genetic factors, specifically *BRCA1* and *BRCA2*, and their role in LR, incidence of a second primary, or contralateral breast disease have not been sufficiently documented as supporting a particular management algorithm. Finally, the concerns and wishes of the patient and her ability to manage the risks of LR must be considered when one discusses treatment options.

Adjunctive Breast Radiation

The role of radiation remains controversial in the management of DCIS patients treated with BCT. Three prospective randomized trials have been performed to evaluate the role of radiation therapy in DCIS patients treated with BCT: National Surgical Adjuvant Breast and Bowel Project (NSABP B-17), European Organization for Research and Treatment of Cancer (EORTC 10853) trial and the UK Coordinating Committee on Cancer Research (UKCCCR) trial.

In 1993, the NSABP reported results of the B-17 trial for a total of 818 women with DCIS who were randomized to BCT or BCT with radiation. After 12 years of follow-up, the cumulative incidence of invasive and noninvasive ipsilateral breast tumor recurrence was 31.7% in the excision alone group and 15.7% in the excision plus radiation therapy group ($P = 0.001$). Overall survival was equivalent in both groups with 86% for excision alone and 87% for patients in the excision plus radiation therapy group ($P = 0.08$). Based on these results it was recommended that excision plus radiation be adopted as the standard of care for treating DCIS patients unless otherwise contraindicated. The results of the B-17 trial remain controversial, as it suggests that all DCIS patients treated with BCT should receive radiation. The trial, however, was not designed to determine whether there is a subset that might be selected to forego radiation.

The EORTC 10853 trial randomly assigned 1,010 patients to evaluate excision alone versus excision plus radiation therapy. With a mean follow-up of only 4.25 years, the LR rates were 17% versus 11%, respectively. Further analysis of the EORTC data revealed that margin status influenced the effect of radiation on LR. There was no statistical difference in LR when margins were free, whereas, when the margins were close or involved, radiation reduced LR from 32% to 16%.

The UKCCCR DCIS trial randomized 1,701 patients to excision ± radiation therapy, as well as ± tamoxifen. The primary outcome for this trial was the incidence of ipsilateral invasive breast cancer. Evaluating only the radiation versus control treatment arms (n = 1030) without tamoxifen, a 16% versus 7% LR was noted for those in the no-radiotherapy arm versus radiation, respectively (P < 0.001). Overall, the majority of patients in these studies had small areas of DCIS (less than 2 cm in diameter) which were radiographically detected. The addition of radiation therapy consistently reduced the risk of recurrent disease in the ipsilateral breast by 40–60%. High-grade DCIS lesions and those with positive margins achieved the greatest benefit from the addition of radiation therapy.

Recent retrospective analysis of over 1,000 patients with DCIS from North America and Europe who were treated with excision and radiation therapy revealed that a margin width of 2 mm combined with radiation achieved excellent local control with 8% LR in 10 years. Prospective trials evaluating BCT ± tamoxifen are being conducted by the Radiation Therapy Oncology Group (RTOG) 98-04 and the Eastern Cooperative Oncology Group (ECOG) E5194.

Role of Chemoprevention: Tamoxifen and Selective Estrogen Receptor Modulators

The nonsteroidal selective estrogen receptor modulator (SERM) tamoxifen has both estrogenic and antiestrogenic effects that are valuable in reducing ipsilateral breast cancer (IBC) and systemic recurrence in estrogen receptor-positive invasive breast cancer patients. The recent NSABP metaanalysis has also demonstrated the reduction of DCIS or invasive contralateral breast cancer (CBC) from 5.1% to 1.9% at 5 years in patients taking tamoxifen. NSABP P-01 prevention trial randomized more than 13,300 high-risk patients to tamoxifen or placebo; a 50% reduction in the incidence of both DCIS and invasive ductal carcinoma was evident for patients receiving tamoxifen. Two prospective randomized trials (NSABP B-24 and UKCCCR) have examined the use of adjuvant tamoxifen in patients with DCIS. NSABP B-24 was a double-blind, prospective, randomized trial for DCIS patients treated with BCT and radiation assigned to either tamoxifen or placebo. Tamoxifen therapy resulted in a consistent reduction in both IBC and CBC; the incidence of all ipsilateral breast recurrences was 11.1% in the placebo arm and 7.7% in the tamoxifen arm after 7 years of follow-up with no statistical difference in overall survival. The cumulative incidence of contralateral breast tumors was 4.9% in the placebo group and 2.3% in the tamoxifen group ($P = 0.01$). In ER positive DCIS patients receiving tamoxifen, there was a relative risk for a breast cancer event of 0.4 ($P < 0.001$). In the ER-negative patients, the relative risk was 0.8 ($P = 0.51$), indicating that the benefit from tamoxifen therapy is limited to the estrogen receptor-positive DCIS patients.

The UKCCCR trial reported the use of tamoxifen in the adjuvant setting for DCIS and excluded patients with positive margins. Ipsilateral events were reduced from 15% in the placebo arm to 13% in the tamoxifen arm. Contralateral events were reduced from 3% to 1%. Overall, the NSABP B-24 study demonstrated a statistically significant reduction in breast cancer recurrence with tamoxifen but no overall difference in survival, whereas the UKCCCR trial found neither a reduction in recurrence nor survival difference, which is potentially explained by the exclusion of patients with positive margins and the older age of patients in the UKCCCR trial.

Tamoxifen therapy is not without risk, especially in postmenopausal women, with at least a twofold increase in endometrial cancer, from a cumulative risk of 5.4 per 1,000 to 13 per 1,000 in patients taking tamoxifen. In addition, thromboembolic events are increased twofold with tamoxifen use compared to control subjects. Raloxifene (Evista) is a second-generation SERM developed specifically to promote bone mineralization and prevent osteoporosis. Its use promotes a favorable lipid profile and does not stimulate endometrial hyperplasia, although the thromboembolic events and menopausal symptoms were similar to those experienced with tamoxifen use. The second chemoprevention trial (NSABP P-2) or STAR trial compared tamoxifen and raloxifene in high-risk postmenopausal women. Recent analysis of the data revealed a reduction in the incidence of invasive ductal carcinoma; however, raloxifene did not significantly reduce the incidence of DCIS. At this time, there are no data that support the use of raloxifene in invasive or noninvasive breast cancer.

IBC recurrence in patients treated with BCT may be considered a complication whose incidence should be limited, as the consequences of an invasive cancer include disease-specific mortality. Approximately 50% of all local failures are invasive disease, and the median time frame of invasive recurrence is nearly 5 years with many invasive recurrences identified at more than 10 years. Most noninvasive recurrences occur within the first 5 years. The treatment of recurrent disease initially treated with BCT performed with adjunctive radiation therapy includes ipsilateral mastectomy with or without axillary sentinel node biopsy, depending on the presence of invasion. If BCT without radiation therapy is the primary treatment, re-excision with adjunctive radiation therapy may be considered depending on the patient's desires and the availability of breast volume. Patients initially treated with lumpectomy alone generally require local re-excision, chest wall irradiation, and possibly chemotherapy. The prognosis for LR after BCT is favorable compared with patients experiencing postmastectomy chest wall recurrence.

The potential deleterious effect of tamoxifen must be considered when this chemopreventive agent is used to further reduce the incidence of recurrence, particularly when the incidence may be already substantially lowered by surgical resection, radiation therapy, or both. Specifically, in postmenopausal women who have retained their uterus, the greater than twofold incidence of endometrial carcinoma and thromboembolic events is a significant complication potential. In patients who are at increased risk for thromboembolic events (atrial fibrillation, history of deep venous thrombosis, history of pulmonary embolus, and relative contraindications of extreme age associated with limited mobility), tamoxifen use is contraindicated.

Outcomes

Total (simple) mastectomy remains the most aggressive and successful surgical treatment for DCIS and the standard against which the outcomes of all other therapies are compared. Long-term follow-up of mastectomy has shown a recurrence rate of 0–2% and disease-specific mortality of 0–1%. Disease-specific mortality is a reflection of unrecognized foci of invasive disease in patients with DCIS. Silverstein evaluated the outcomes of invasive LR after BCT for patients with DCIS. The 8-year probability of local invasive cancer in a cohort of 707 patients was 9.3%, and the probability of breast cancer-specific mortality rate was 2.1%. For patients who developed an invasive recurrence, the disease-specific mortality rate was 14.1% with a distant recurrence rate of 27.1%. The median time to noninvasive cancer recurrence was 22 months and 58 months for invasive LR. Overall, the majority of DCIS patients that recur can be salvaged; however, in the small group of patients who do recur with an invasive breast cancer, the survival is reduced to 85%.

Selected Readings

Anderson BO, Calhoun KE, Rosen EL (2006) Evolving con-Burstein HJ, Kornelia P, Wong JS, et al. (2004) Ductal cepts in the management of lobular neoplasia. J Natl carcinoma in situ of the breast. NEJM 350:1430–1441 Cancer Instit 4:511–522

Chuba PJ, Hamre MR, Yap J, et al. (2005) Bilateral risk for subsequent breast cancer after lobular carcinoma in situ: Analysis of surveillance, epidemiology, and end results Data. J Clin Onc 23:5534–5531

Fisher B, Dignam J, Wolmark N, et al. (1999) Tamoxifen in treatment of intraductal breast cancer: National Surgical Adjuvant Breast and Bowel Project B-24 randomised controlled trial. Lancet 353:1993

Holland PA, Gandhi A, Knox WF, et al. (1998) The importance of complete excision in the presentation of local recurrence of ductal carcinoma in situ. BR J Cancer 77:110

Leonard GD, Swain SM (2004) Ductal carcinoma in situ: complexities and challenges. J Natl Cancer Inst 96:906–920

Li CI, Malone KE, Saltzman BS, Daling JR (2006) Risk of invasive breast carcinoma among women diagnosed with ductal carcinoma in situ and lobular carcinoma in situ, 1988–2001. Cancer 106:2104–2112

Page DL, Lagios MD, Jensen RA (2004) In situ carcinoma of the breast. Bland KI, Copeland EM, eds. The Breast, 3rd edn. W. B. Saunders, Philadelphia

Romero L, Klein L, Ye W, et al. (2004) Outcome after invasive recurrence in patients with ductal carcinoma in situ of the breast. Am J Surg 188:371–376

Silverstein MJ (2003) The University of Southern California/ Van Nuys prognostic index for ductal carcinoma in situ of the breast. Am J Surg 186:337–343

Vogel VG, Costantino JP, Wickerham DL, et al. (2006) Effects of tamoxifen vs. raloxifene on the risk of developing invasive breast cancer and other disease outcomes. JAMA 295:2727–2926

5
Breast Carcinoma: Stages I and II

Emma L. Murray and J. Michael Dixon

Pearls and Pitfalls

- Invasive cancer is increasing in frequency as a result of more extensive screening, an increasingly elderly population, social trends, later first pregnancy, and increasing use of hormone replacement therapy (HRT).
- Mammographic screening reduces breast cancer mortality in women aged from 50–70 years by 40%.
- In operable stage I and II breast cancer survival rates for breast conserving surgery (BCS) are equivalent to those for mastectomy.
- Breast conserving surgery is suitable for the majority of patients with cancers under 4 cm and excision margins > 1 mm have not been shown to decrease local recurrence but do adversely affect cosmetic outcome.
- Mastectomy is favored for patients who: (i) choose mastectomy; (ii) have multiple cancers; (iii) have large areas of non-invasive disease or, (iv) where BCS would leave an unacceptable cosmetic result (most cancers over 4 cm).
- All patients with invasive cancer should have axillary nodes removed and examined histologically but axillary dissection should be limited to patients with involved axillary nodes or at high risk of axillary lymph node involvement.
- Patients with involved axillary nodes should have axillary node dissection (AND) or axillary radiotherapy.

K.I. Bland et al. (eds.), *Surgery in Breast Cancer and Melanoma*, DOI 10.1007/978-1-84996-435-7_5,
© Springer-Verlag London Limited 2011

- Patients having BCS for invasive cancer should have whole breast radiotherapy with a local boost in younger patients (< 60 years).
- Patients at high risk of local recurrence after mastectomy benefit from chest wall radiotherapy which lowers rates of local recurrence and improves survival.
- For patients with Estrogen and/or progesterone receptor positive invasive breast cancer (ER/PgR) hormonal therapy should be considered.
- Chemotherapy significantly decreases rates of local recurrence, particularly in young women.
- The addition of Herceptin in high risk patients with HER2 positive cancers reduces recurrence by 50%.
- Patients with large operable or locally advanced breast cancer (LABC) can be given neoadjuvant therapy to shrink large tumor to permit less extensive surgery or allow a LABC to become operable.
- Although neoadjuvant chemotherapy is most commonly used, neoadjuvant endocrine therapy is an option for post-menopausal women with large ER rich cancers.

Introduction

Epidemiology, Risk Factors and Genetics

Over one million new cases of invasive breast cancer are diagnosed worldwide each year. Breast cancer is the commonest malignancy in women and comprises 18% of female cancers. The incidence is increasing and affects one in eight women in major Western countries.

The incidence of breast cancer increases with age, doubling every 10 years until the menopause, when the rate of increase slows. Age adjusted incidence and mortality vary between countries but, these differences are starting to diminish. In migrants from East to West the rates of breast cancer assume the rate in the host country within one or two generations, indicating that environmental factors are of greater importance than genetic factors.

A strong genetic predisposition accounts for up to 10% of breast cancer in Western countries. Two well documented genes, BRCA1 and 2, located on the long arms of chromosomes 17 and 13, respectively, account for a substantial proportion of high risk families. Although rare the p53 and PTEN genes are associated with familial cancer syndromes that include a high risk of breast cancer. A few families are described in which multiple cases of breast cancer are attributed to mutations in ATM and Chk2. There are likely to be other, as yet unidentified, contributory genes. The criteria for identifying women at substantially increased risk based on their family history, who may be eligible for genetic testing and screening from a young age, can be seen in Table 5.1.

TABLE 5.1. Criteria for identifying women at risk of breast cancer.

Familial breast cancer – criteria for identifying women at substantially increased risk

The following categories identify women who have three or more times the population risk of developing breast cancer

A woman who has:

One first degree* relative with bilateral breast cancer or breast and ovarian cancer or

One first degree relative with breast cancer diagnosed under the age of 40 years or one first degree male relative with breast cancer diagnosed at any age or

Two first or second degree relatives with breast cancer diagnosed under the age of 60 years or ovarian cancer at any age on the same side of the family or

Three first or second relatives with breast and ovarian cancer on the same side of the family

Criteria for identifying women at very high risk in whom gene testing might be appropriate

Families with four or more relatives affected with either breast or ovarian cancer in three generations and one alive affected individual

*First degree relative is mother, sister, or daughter. Second degree female relative is grandmother, granddaughter, aunt, or niece.

Women who have proliferative breast changes, in particular atypical epithelial hyperplasia, have four to five times the risk of developing breast cancer. Other benign pathologies including, palpable cysts, complex fibroadenoma, ductal papilloma, sclerosing adenosis and, florid epithelial hyperplasia have a slightly higher, but not clinically significant, risk of breast cancer. Ionizing radiation, particularly mantle radiotherapy given at a young age for Hodgkin's Lymphoma, increases a woman's risk, warranting early screening.

Early menarche, late menopause, nulliparity and late first pregnancy increase the risk of developing breast cancer, as do combined HRT preparations given after the menopause (Table 5.2).

TABLE 5.2. Established and probable risk factors for breast cancer.

Factor	Relative risk	High risk group
Age	>10	Elderly
Geographical location	5	Developed country
Age at menarche	3	Before age 11
Age at menopause	2	After age 54
Age at first full pregnancy	3	First child in early 40s
Family history	>2	Breast cancer in first degree relative when young
Previous benign disease	4–5	Atypical hyperplasia
Cancer in other breast	4	
Socioeconomic group	2	Groups I and II
Diet	1.5	High intake of saturated fat
Premenopausal	0.7	BMI > 35
Postmenopausal	2	BMI > 35
Alcohol consumption	1.3	Excessive intake

(continued)

Table 5.2. (continued)

Factor	Relative risk	High risk group
Exposure to ionising radiation	3	Abnormal exposure in young females > 10 years of age
Taking exogenous hormones		
Oral contraceptives	1.24	Current use
Combined hormone replacement therapy	2.3	Use for > 10 years
Unopposed estrogen	1.3	Use for > 10 years
Diethylstilbestrol	2	Use during pregnancy

Clinical Presentation and Preoperative Evaluation and Diagnosis

Women with breast cancer either present symptomatically to breast clinics or are diagnosed through screening programs. All patients referred to a breast clinic or identified with a suspicious lesion through screening should undergo triple assessment, a combination of clinical examination, imaging and core biopsy, fine needle aspiration cytology (FNAC) or both. In centers with large volumes triple assessment can be undertaken in a one stop clinic.

Clinical Examination

Inspection of both breasts should take place in a good light with the patient's hands by her side, above her head and finally, on her hips. Skin dimpling is present in up to 25% of patients with a palpable underling tumour but can be secondary to surgery, trauma or benign pathology.

Palpation of the breasts should be performed with the patient lying flat with her arms above her head. This makes abnormal areas easier to define. The tissues are palpated with the fingertips. If a discrete lesion is found its contour, texture and degree of deep fixation to the pectoral muscles must be documented. The lesion should be measured with callipers and a diagram documenting any abnormalities recorded. The axillary and supraclavicular nodes should be checked but, clinical assessment of these is inaccurate.

Mammography

Mammography is performed on symptomatic women over 35 years of age. Below this age the breast tissues are radiodense and mammography is of limited value. It should only be performed in younger women if a strong clinical suspicion of a cancer exists. Mammography performed every 2–3 years from the age of 50 is also a proven method of breast screening and reduces subsequent mortality by 40%. Two views, oblique and craniocaudal are obtained to allow detection of mass lesions, parenchymal distortion and, microcalcifications.

Ultrasound

In women under the age of 35 years breast ultrasonography (US) is the most useful imaging modality. In older women it can be used to further define localized palpable and mammographic lesions. High frequency sound waves are beamed through the breast and reflections are detected and turned into images. Cancers usually have indistinct outlines and are hypoechoic.

MRI

Magnetic resonance imaging (MRI) is not in routine clinical use but is an accurate way of imaging the breast. Its sensitivity for cancer is high and it is valuable in demonstrating the extent of invasive and non-invasive disease. Its role in improving the success rate of BCS procedures is currently being evaluated. It has proven to be a valuable screening tool for high risk women between the ages of 35 and 50 and is the optimum method for imaging breast implants.

Breast Biopsy

Core Biopsy

Core biopsy is preferable to FNAC because it allows differentiation between invasive and non-invasive carcinoma. Local anesthetic containing adrenaline is infiltrated around the tumor and through a small skin incision cores of tissue are removed from the mass or area of ultrasonic/ mammographic abnormality, by means of a 14 gauge needle combined with a mechanical gun. Multiple cores are taken to ensure adequate sampling of all parts of the lesion so that its nature can be classified.

Fine Needle Aspiration Cytology (FNAC)

If clinical examination and or imaging confirm a suspicion of malignancy, a breast biopsy is required. Aspiration of solid lesions aims to obtain enough cells for cytological analysis. Image guidance increases accuracy in small and impalpable lesions. Results can be made available within the hour.

Classification of Invasive Breast Cancers

Breast cancer is derived from the epithelial cells that line the terminal duct lobular unit. An invasive breast cancer is one in which there is dissemination of cancer cells outside the basement membrane of the ducts and lobules into the surrounding adjacent normal tissue.

The most commonly used classification of invasive breast cancer divides them into ductal and lobular types. This classification was based on the belief that ductal carcinoma in situ arose from ducts and lobular carcinoma from lobules. It is clear that both invasive ductal and lobular cancers arise from the terminal duct lobular unit so this terminology is no longer appropriate but remains in common use.

Some tumors show distinct patterns of growth and cellular morphology and on this basis certain types of breast cancer can be identified. Those with special features are called invasive carcinomas of special type whereas the remainder are considered to be of no special type. Certain special type tumors have a much better prognosis than tumors which are of no special type (Fig. 5.1). So called invasive lobular carcinomas (ILC) can be difficult to diagnose because their pattern of single file cell infiltration does not form a well defined mass lesion clinically or on imaging.

Prognostic information, among tumors of no special type, can be gained by grading the tumor differentiation. Degrees of glandular formation, nuclear pleomorphism, frequency and mitosis are scored from 1–3. These values are combined and converted into three groups; grade 1 (scores 3–5), grade 2 (scores 6 and 7) and, grade 3 (scores 8 and 9). This derived grade is an important predictor of both disease free and overall survival. Histological evidence of lymphatic or vascular

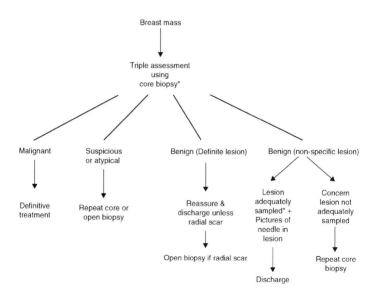

FIGURE 5.1. Triple assessment biopsy procedures.
*A minimum of 3–5 cores is required to be certain that the lesion is adequately sampled.

invasion (LVI) is associated with an increased risk of local and systemic recurrence.

The introduction of molecular diagnostics has heralded a change in the way in which breast cancer is reported. Markers including Estrogen receptor (ER), progesterone receptor (PgR) and HER2 status are now reported routinely.

Staging of Invasive Tumors

Two staging classifications are commonly applied to breast cancer but, neither are well suited to the disease. The tumor node metastases (TNM) system depends on clinical measurements and clinical assessment of lymph node status, both of which are inaccurate. The International Union Against Cancer (UICC) system incorporates the TNM classification. To improve the TNM classification a separate system of pathological classification has been included to allow tumor size and node status, as assessed by the pathologist, to be taken into account. Prognosis and treatment relate to the stage of the disease at presentation (Tables 5.3 and 5.4).

Most patients with operable or early breast cancer require only a limited series of pre-operative investigations. A full blood count, liver function tests and a chest radiograph are usually performed. Small cancers have a low incidence of

TABLE 5.3. Classification of invasive breast cancers.

Special types	No special type (NST)
• Classic lobular	Classic ductal*
• Tubular	
• Mucoid/mucinous	
• Cribriform	
• Papillary	
• Medullary	
• Classic lobular	

*Useful prognostic information can be obtained by grading such cancers.

TABLE 5.4. TNM and UICC classifications of breast cancer.

TNM classification of breast tumors

Tis Cancer in situ	N0 No regional lymph node metastases
T1 < 2 cm (T1a < 0.5 cm, T1b > 0.5–1 cm, T1c 1–2 cm)	N1 Palpable mobile involved ipsilateral axillary nodes
T2 > 2–5 cm	N2 Fixed involved ipsilateral axillary nodes
T3 > 5 cm	N3 Ipsilateral internal mammary node involvement (rarely clinically detectable)
T4a Involvement of chest wall	M0 No evidence of metastases
T4b Involvement of skin (ulceration, direct infiltration, peau d'orange, and satellite nodules)	M1 Distant metastases (includes ipsilateral supraclavicular nodes)
T4c T4a and T4b together	
T4d Inflammatory cancer	

Correlation of UICC (1987) and TNM Classification of tumors

TNM classification	UICC stage
T1, N0, M0	I
T1, N1, M0; T2, N0–1, M0	II
Any T, N2–3, M0; T3, any N, M0; T4, any N, M0	III
Any T, any N, M1	IV

systemic spread and if all initial blood investigations and the chest radiograph are normal no further investigations are required. If there are localized symptoms or any abnormality in these tests, liver and bone scans should be undertaken.

Options for Stage 1 and 2 Breast Cancer

Most patients with operable, stage I and II, breast cancer benefit from a combination of local treatment, to control local disease and, systemic treatment to combat potential metastatic disease.

The aim of local treatment is to achieve long term local disease control with the minimum of local morbidity. Local treatments consist of surgery and radiotherapy. Surgery can be excision of the tumor with surrounding normal tissue (BCS) or mastectomy.

Surgical Options and Selection for Therapy

At least 12 randomized clinical trials have compared mastectomy and BCS and shown a non significant reduction in death in favor of BCS. Local recurrence rates are similar with a non significant but lower rate of recurrence in favor of mastectomy. Two large randomized trials comparing mastectomy and BCS have shown no significant differences in survival after 20 years of follow up.

Patients suitable for breast conserving surgery are those with:

- Single clinical and mammographic lesions
- Tumors staged as T1, T2 < 4 cm, N0, N1, M0
- Tumors > 4 cm in a large breast

  Patients suitable for mastectomy are:

- Those who prefer treatment by mastectomy
- Those for whom BCS would produce an unacceptable cosmetic result
- Those with multifocal or multicentric operable breast cancer

Operative Management

Breast Conservation Surgery

Breast conserving surgery aims to excise the tumor and any surrounding ductal carcinoma in-situ (DCIS) with a 1 cm margin of macroscopically normal tissue (wide local excision (WLE).

Impalpable lesions can be localized preoperatively by a number of techniques. The most common involves insertion of an image guided hook wire to localize the cancer, with surgical dissection being directed by the wire.

There is no size limit for BCS. Extensive excisions of the tumor bearing breast quadrant (quadrantectomy) were performed in the past. Quadrantic and segmental excisions are no longer favored as they do not significantly lower local recurrence rates and, are associated with poorer cosmetic outcomes. Up to 10% of the breast volume can be removed without serious adverse cosmetic effect. Adequate excision of lesions measuring over 4 cm are generally associated with poor cosmesis. For this reason, in most breast units BCS tends to be limited to lesions of less than 4 cm. Women with large breasts are the exception to this rule as BCS for tumors in excess of 4 cm may still be possible with good cosmesis, particularly if combined with a reduction/oncoplastic approach.

Complete excision of all invasive and in-situ disease is essential. Intra-operative specimen radiography can help to confirm excision of the lesion with any associated DCIS and improve the rate of complete excision. A negative margin of 1–2 mm is adequate. Wider margins do not reduce local recurrence further but do adversely affect cosmesis.

Local recurrence is on average 3.4 times more likely if margins are involved. Neither atypical ductal hyperplasia (ADH) nor lobular carcinoma at the margins necessitates re-excision as these histological features do not increase the rate of recurrence. Those factors associated with an increased risk of local recurrence are listed in Table 5.5.

Mastectomy

Around one third of patients with localized symptomatic breast cancers are unsuitable for BCS. A further number of women, suitable for BCS, opt for more radical surgery. These patients can be treated by mastectomy. The aim of mastectomy is to remove as much breast tissue as is possible, with some overlying skin and, usually the nipple. The breast is

TABLE 5.5. Risk factors for local recurrence of breast cancer.

Risk factors for local recurrence of cancer after breast conservation

Factor	Relative risk
Involved margins	X 3–5
Extensive in-situ component	X 3
Patient's age (<35) (vs. > 50)	X 3
Lymphatic or vascular invasion	X 2
Histological grade II or III (vs. I)	X 1.5

Factors associated with local recurrence after mastectomy

Axillary lymph node involvement

Lymphatic or vascular invasion by cancer

Grade III carcinoma

Tumor over 4 cm in diameter (pathological)

removed from the chest wall muscles (pectoralis major and minor, rectus abdominis and serratus anterior) but these muscles, their nerve supplies and the pectoral fascia are left intact.

The Axilla

Breast conserving surgery and mastectomy, for early stage invasive breast cancer, need to be combined with an axillary node procedure. The axilla receives approximately 95% of the breast. The axillary nodes lie below the axillary vein and, can be divided into three groups in relation to the pectoralis minor muscle. Level I nodes lie lateral to the muscle; level II (central) nodes lie behind the muscle and, level III (apical) lie between the medial border, the first rib and the axillary vein. The remaining 5% of lymph from the breast cancer drains via the internal mammary and intercostals routes.

Up to 40% of patients with early invasive breast cancer have involvement of the axillary nodes at diagnosis. Axillary lymph node status is the most significant prognostic factor in patients with breast cancer. Evaluation of axillary lymph node status is therefore critical for accurately staging patients and provides a basis for making decisions on management and treatment. Both the number and level of involved nodes predict survival.

Clinical and radiological prediction of lymph node involvement are unreliable but routine ultrasound scan of the axilla followed by FNAC or core biopsy of suspicious nodes can detect up to 40% of patients with axillary node involvement prior to surgery.

Axillary Surgery

Axillary surgery can be used both to stage and to treat the axilla. Standard histopathological examination of excised nodes is essential and histological involvement is of greater prognostic significance than metastases seen only using immunohistochemical techniques.

Staging the Axilla

Lymphatic drainage from the breast occurs sequentially so the status of the first node directly draining the primary lesion predicts the node status of the remaining nodes in the axilla. This first draining node is called the sentinel node. Identification of the sentinel node is possible via peritumoral, intradermal or, subareolar injection of blue dye (isosulfan blue or patent blue V) and radioactive colloid. Histological assessment of the blue and or radioactive nodes, predicts node status with over 95% accuracy. In reality few patients have a single sentinel node, the average being between 2 and 3, with 25% of metastases being in neither the bluest nor hottest node. Some patients with axillary nodal metastases have no sentinel nodes because lymphatic flow is blocked as a consequence of nodal involvement. The false negative rate is low at less than 5% in experienced hands and can be reduced further by removing any palpable suspicious nodes in addition to the nodes which are blue or radioactive.

Sentinel node biopsy (SNB) can be performed as an out-patient or as a day case procedure. It is now standard practice for patients with clinically and ultrasonographically N0 tumors, particularly those with tumors < 2 cm, in whom the likelihood of nodal involvement is low. The value of preoperative scintigraphy is unclear. It identifies drainage to the internal mammary nodes, but metastasis to these nodes alone is rare. A few centers use blue dye alone and combine this procedure with dissection of palpable nodes (axillary node sampling (ANS)) and claim results equivalent to SNB. Prior to SNB surgical removal of levels I and II or levels I, II and III, so called axillary node dissection (AND) or clearance (ANC), was standard practice. Such extensive axillary dissection should now be limited to patients with evidence of axillary node involvement or who are highly likely to have involved nodes.

Trials comparing SNB with AND have shown that the former produces less morbidity (decreased sensory loss and arm swelling) and shortens hospital stay. Routine axillary dissection with its morbidities cannot be supported particularly in low risk groups. Where the sentinel node or axillary sampling reveal that the nodes are not involved no further treatment is required to the axilla.

Treatment of Axillary Disease

If pre-operative biopsy or ANS or SNB demonstrate metastatic disease, then either complete AND (levels I and II if disease at level I or I, II and III if disease at level II) or axillary radiotherapy is recommended. Surgery and radiotherapy are both effective and are associated with similar survival rates. Surgical dissection offers a lower rate of axillary recurrence and radiotherapy cannot be repeated. Although recurrence rates following complete AND are low the morbidity of the procedure is high.

Studies are ongoing to ascertain the need for axillary therapy where only isolated micro metastases present in the SNB. A watch and wait policy with no surgical staging procedure has been advocated for some patients with low risk invasive cancers but, until the results from studies are available some form of axillary surgery should be considered for all patients with breast cancer.

Postoperative Management

Drains are not necessary following BCS. They do not protect against hematoma formation and increase infection rates. They are used routinely following mastectomy and axillary surgery. The optimal time for drain removal remains a matter of controversy. In the majority of units drains will either be removed when draining below a specified volume, i.e. 30 ml in 24 h or, after a maximal period of time, i.e. 5 days, after which time they pose a considerable infection risk.

Complications of Breast Surgery

Bleeding with resultant hematoma is a not an uncommon problem with the routine use of low molecular weight heparins and occurs in 2–3% of patients.

Infection after breast surgery is reported in up to 10% of patients. When it occurs after mastectomy it is usually secondary to flap necrosis or infection entering through the drain site or after seroma aspiration. Treatment is with antibiotics and, if required aspiration and irrigation of any infected cavity, using local anesthetic for irrigation. Formal opening of the mastectomy wound with packing of the cavity is rarely required and when required often results in an ugly, contracted scar. There is no consensus on the use of prophylactic antibiotics to reduce rates of wound infection after surgery for breast cancer. One meta-analysis did show a significant reduction in infection rate after a single pre-operative dose of antibiotic.

Seroma affects a third to a half of all mastectomy patients and, is a common complication of breast surgery. Collection of inflammatory fluid occurs under the mastectomy flaps after the suction drains have been removed. It is more common after mastectomy and ANC than after mastectomy and SNB or ANS. The rate of seroma formation may be reduced by "quilting", a process of securing the flaps to the chest wall with rows of absorbable sutures. Treatment of seroma includes recurrent needle aspiration or simply observation, as most resolve given time.

Incomplete tumor excision following BCS affects 15–20% of women, with higher rates seen in lobular cancers. Re-excision of the positive margins or mastectomy is often necessary in these patients.

Morbidity of Axillary Treatments

Nerve damage is a common complication following axillary surgery and is more common during AND than with SNB or ANS. Preservation of the intercostobrachial nerve can avoid numbness and paresthesia down the upper inner arm. Brachial plexopathy can occur secondary to overlapping radiotherapy fields, but with careful planning is now avoidable.

Wound infection of the axilla affects between 5% and 10% of patients and is more prevalent following AND than with lesser procedures. Seroma occur in 50% of patients following AND but in only 5% following SNB or ANS. The rate of seroma formation appears to be reduced by quilting the axillary skin to the chest wall.

A reduced range of shoulder movement and occasionally a frozen shoulder is evident following either surgery or radiotherapy. Regular post treatment exercise under the guidance of a physiotherapist minimize these.

Lymphoedema affects up to 10% of patients following AND to level II or III. The effects are worse when extensive axillary surgery and radiotherapy are combined. Radiotherapy should not be given following a level III dissection. The most dramatic lymphoedema is produced by axillary recurrence. There is no curative treatment for lymphoedema and therapy remains symptomatic.

Aesthetic and Hospital Stay Considerations

The majority of BCS procedures are performed under general anesthesia, as day case procedures. It is possible to perform BCS under local anesthesia allowing those unfit for general anesthesia to still have BCS.

Cosmetic Outcomes and BCS

Women who have a satisfactory cosmetic outcome following BCS are less anxious and depressed. They have better body image, freedom of dress, sexuality and self-esteem. Poor cosmetic outcome affects at least 17% of women, following BCS and radiotherapy.

The most important determinant of cosmesis is the volume of tissue excised, both primarily and on re-excision. Large volume (>10%) excisions and excision of skin, are associated with worse outcomes. Skin should be excised only if directly involved by the underlying tumor. Options for patients with large or central tumors include neoadjuvant systemic therapy to shrink the tumor, an oncoplastic procedure to displace or transfer tissue into the breast defect, or surgery (usually a breast reduction) to the opposite breast to obtain symmetry.

Controversy has surrounded which incisions give the best cosmetic results. Scars placed parallel both to the lines of maximum resting skin tension (Kraissl's lines) and parallel to the orientation of collagen fibers (Langer's lines) heal most rapidly, produce the best cosmetic incisions and have the least incidence of hypertrophy and keloid formation (Fig. 5.2). Circumareolar incisions for excision of cancers, close to the nipple and submammary incisions for cancers in the lower half of the breast produce excellent cosmetic results. Excisions in the upper outer quadrant tend to be associated with better outcomes than those in other quadrants. Limiting the length

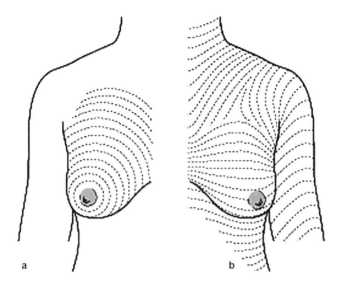

FIGURE 5.2. The direction of (**a**) Langer's lines and (**b**) Kraissl's dynamic lines of maximum resting skin tension (Reprinted from Dixon JM, 2006a).

of incision is important to enhance cosmesis. To minimize distortion, the breast tissue should be mobilized and closure of the defect undertaken in a layered fashion with absorbable sutures, finishing with an absorbable subcuticular skin closure.

Cosmetic outcome tends to be better where BCS is undertaken on moderately sized breasts. Cosmesis is adversely affected by a post-operative complication such as hematoma, seroma or infection. Axillary clearance procedures can also worsen cosmetic outcome by causing breast edema. Radiotherapy causes fibrosis and unsightly skin changes.

Breast Reconstruction Following Mastectomy

The majority of patients undergoing mastectomy should be considered for breast reconstruction. Immediate reconstruction produces better aesthetic outcomes and has psychological advantages over delayed reconstruction. There is no evidence that reconstruction increases the rate or delays detection of local recurrence. Options include the use of implants, tissue expanders, combined expander implant devices and the use of myocutaneous flaps.

The most common flaps are based on the latissimus dorsi muscle (LD flap) or transverse rectus abdominis muscle (TRAM flap) both of which can be harvested with or without their overlying fat and skin. Myocutaneous flaps with or without an implant produce the most natural looking breast mounds. The LD flap more often requires an implant to achieve adequate volume. Flaps can be pedicled (left attached to their blood supply) or free (re-anastomosed to a new blood supply after transfer). It is possible to limit the amount of muscle weakness in TRAM flaps by raising the flap on the blood vessels and dissecting these out from the muscle. This is known as the di-ep flap because the blood vessels dissected out are the deep inferior epigastric vessels which are then anastomosed to the axillary or internal mammary vessels to create the new breast mound. The nipple can be reconstructed later by various techniques. This is usually undertaken 3–6 months after the initial breast reconstruction to allow the breast to settle (Fig. 5.3).

Radiotherapy has a deleterious effect on all reconstructions, particularly when implants are used. Women requiring adjuvant chest wall radiotherapy following mastectomy, based on their risk factors, must be fully informed of the pros and cons of immediate and delayed reconstruction and the potential detrimental effects of radiotherapy. In such women a technique without an implant is favored if immediate reconstruction is chosen.

Complications following Breast Reconstruction

The most common complication after the use of prostheses is the formation and subsequent contraction of fibrous capsules around the implants. Capsular contracture results

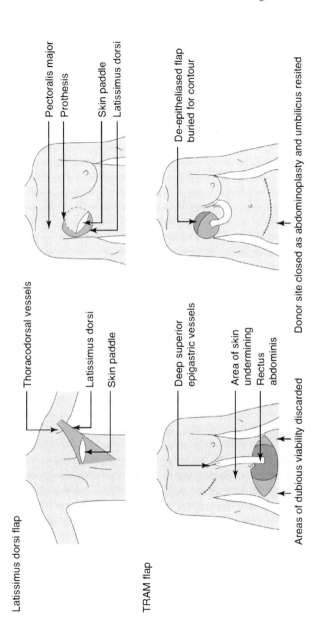

FIGURE 5.3. Breast reconstruction with myocutaneous flaps. The TRAM flap is shown as a pedicled flap but is most frequently performed as a free flap. (Reprinted from Dixon JM, 2006b).

in hardening, distortion and an unfavorable cosmetic appearance of the breast mound, and requires revisional surgery. Infection can be a problem, particularly in LD flaps if an implant is inserted. This results in removal of the prosthesis. Up to 50% of patients get back wound seromas with LD flaps but the frequency can be reduced by suturing the skin flaps to the underlying muscle (quilting). The greatest problem with free flaps, such as the TRAM flap is necrosis of skin and fat. Major necrosis occurs in up to 10% of patients who have pedicled TRAM flaps, but affects fewer than 5% of patients with free TRAM flaps. Radiotherapy increases the risk of fat necrosis. Abdominal weakness and abdominal herniae are also common problems after TRAM flaps.

Role of Radiotherapy

All patients should receive radiotherapy following BCS. This reduces the rate of local recurrence and may improve survival. A top up boost of 10–20 Gy given to the tumor bed following whole breast radiotherapy, further reduces local recurrence in all age groups, but with only small absolute benefit to those over 60 years of age. In the older age group, if all margins are clear it appears boost radiotherapy may be omitted. As yet, it has not been possible to identify patients who do not require radiotherapy. Several new techniques of partial breast radiotherapy, delivered using standard equipment, given intraoperatively or through a catheter inserted at operation are being evaluated. Results to date have indicted excellent local control rates.

Following mastectomy, patients with a high risk of local recurrence benefit from postoperative radiotherapy to the chest wall, as do women with pectoral muscle involvement or, risk factors including multiple node involvement. There is a three-fold reduction in local recurrence at 15 years combining radiotherapy. The most significant difference is in the first 5 years.

Complications Following Radiotherapy

Increasingly sophisticated machines and smaller fractions have led to a minimization of skin dosing. This is reflected in the reducing number of immediate skin reactions and subsequent telangiectasia. Tangential fields now include only a portion of the left anterior descending coronary artery and a small fraction of lung tissue in the irradiated field. Previous radiotherapy techniques were responsible for large dosing to the heart and for a number of cardiac deaths, many years after treatment. Radiation pneumonitis, usually transient, has been minimized by tangential field radiotherapy and affects less than 2% of patients. Rib doses and therefore damage are also now much less common. Pain in the treated area remains a problem for some patients and is possibly caused by localized vasculitis.

Role of Systemic Therapy

Adjuvant Use of Systemic Therapy

Systemic therapy improves survival of patients with early breast cancer. More than half of patients with operable breast cancer who undergo locoregional treatment alone die from metastatic disease. This suggests that micro metastases are present at diagnosis. The only way to improve survival is to give systemic medical treatment. Systemic treatment can be given as endocrine, chemo or targeted therapy. It may be given after (adjuvant) or before (neoadjuvant) locoregional treatment.

Adjuvant Endocrine Therapy

Adjuvant endocrine therapies are only effective in patients with ER or PgR positive disease. Until recently tamoxifen was the most commonly used agent in this setting for both pre and post menopausal women. Tamoxifen is a partial Estrogen antagonist but has agonist affects on endometrium, lipids and bone. When given for 5 years it has been shown to reduce the risk of contralateral breast cancer by 40–50% (Table 5.6). It may be less effective against HER2 positive tumors.

The third generation selective aromatase inhibitors (AI's) anastrozole, letrozole and exemestane, are a major development in adjuvant therapy for postmenopausal women with early breast cancer. They show superiority to tamoxifen in postmenopausal women. They act by blocking the synthesis of Estrogen, mediated through the aromatase enzyme. They have been shown to improve disease free and metastatic free survival and, to a greater degree than tamoxifen. They reduce the risk of contralateral breast cancer by a further 40–50% compared to tamoxifen.

Data from the first trial to compare tamoxifen with anastrozole (The ATAC trial-Arimidex, Tamoxifen Alone or in Combination) in over 9,000 women, demonstrated a significant disease free survival benefit with anastrozole compared with tamoxifen. Trials have since shown the benefit of letrozole over tamoxifen as first line treatment and also of switching after tamoxifen given for 2–3 years of treatment to anastrozole or exemestane for 2–3 years compared to taking 5 years of tamoxifen alone. Further evidence consistent with the effectiveness of these drugs comes from the Canadian

TABLE 5.6. Proportional risk reductions after 5 years of tamoxifen by age group after exclusion of patients with Estrogen receptor poor disease.

Age (years)	% Proportion of Estrogen receptor positive patients	% Proportional reduction (SD) in annual odds	
		Recurrence	Death
<50	92	45 (8)	32 (10)
50–59	93	37 (6)	11 (8)
60–69	95	54 (5)	33 (6)
>70	94	54 (13)	34 (13)
All	94	47 (3)	26 (4)

led MA17 trial. This revealed that letrozole, when given following 5 years of tamoxifen, reduces risks of local recurrence in ER positive, node negative and positive patients, and produces a significant survival benefit in patients with node positive disease. Current options for post menopausal women are therefore 5 years of tamoxifen alone, 5 years of anastrozole or letrozole, 2–3 years of tamoxifen followed by 2–3 years of anastrozole or exemestane or 5 years of tamoxifen followed by 5 years of letrozole.

In premenopausal women with hormone sensitive disease options include tamoxifen or tamoxifen combined with ovarian ablation, most commonly using a gonadotrophin releasing hormone analogue such as goserelin. The addition of tamoxifen to goserelin appears to improve survival in women with ER positive disease. What is not clear yet is whether benefit is to be gained from adding goserelin to tamoxifen. Trials are underway to compare goserelin and tamoxifen to goserelin and an aromatase inhibitor.

Adjuvant Chemotherapy

The benefits of chemotherapy are greatest in women up to the age of 70 years (Table 5.7). Chemotherapy does not only produce its effects through the induction of amenorrhea. Currently increasing tumor size, involved nodes, Estrogen receptor negativity, HER2 positivity, presence of LVI and, the age of the patient (<35 years) are factors considered when deciding the need for and type of chemotherapy. Chemotherapy does not seem to produce substantial benefits in postmenopausal women with grade I or II, ER rich, HER2 negative breast cancer who receive appropriate endocrine therapy.

Anthracycline containing combinations that use doxorubicin or epirubicin are more effective than traditional CMF combinations and are now standard. The addition of taxanes to anthracyclines further improves survival in node positive disease, over anthracyclines alone. With new treatment regimens, five year survival in node positive women has risen from 65% to over 85% (Table 5.7).

TABLE 5.7. Reduction in recurrence and mortality in trials of polychemotherapy (From Early Breast Cancer Trialists' Collaborative Group, 1998).

Age (years)	% Reduction (SD) in annual odds of recurrence	% Reduction (SD) in odds of death
<40	37 (7)	27 (8)
40–49	34 (5)	27 (5)
50–59	22 (4)	14 (4)
60–69	18 (4)	8 (4)
All	23 (8)	15 (2)

Combinations of Chemotherapy and Hormonal Therapy

The use of chemotherapy and tamoxifen in combination is more effective than either alone, for women with high risk ER positive cancer. Efficacy is greater when tamoxifen is given after chemotherapy, rather than concurrently. No data exist on whether the same is true of ovarian ablation or AI's, but it would seem prudent to assume so.

A recent study suggested that for those patients under the age of 40 years, who remain amenorrheic following chemotherapy, prognosis is better. This raises the possibility that ovarian suppression may be beneficial after chemotherapy in patients with ER positive cancer whose menses persist.

Trastuzumab

The transmembrane growth factor receptor HER2 is associated with a poor prognosis and, is expressed in around 20% of all cancers. Trastuzumab is a humanized monoclonal antibody against the external domain of the receptor, with clinical affect against tumors expressing HER2. Trials have shown that it reduces recurrence by 50% when used in the adjuvant setting in patients with early breast cancer. Lapatinib, a HER1 and HER2 tyrosine kinase inhibitor, is also effective in HER2 positive cancer and is currently being evaluated in trials.

Neoadjuvant Use of Systemic Therapy

Neoadjuvant treatment was initially given to patients with locally advanced, inoperable breast cancers but its use has been extended to patients with early, operable breast cancer. The aim in this setting is to downstage cancers, to allow BCS.

Neoadjuvant Chemotherapy

Neoadjuvant chemotherapy achieves clinical regression of tumors in 70–80% of patients. This suggests that early breast cancers are more chemosensitive than metastatic disease. Complete pathological response is seen in up to 20% of patients, particularly in Estrogen receptor negative patients. Complete response is a predictor of better long-term outcome.

Trials have shown equivalence in survival between neoadjuvant and adjuvant regimens, when the chemotherapy regimens are similar in composition. The advantages of neoadjuvant therapy are tumor downstaging to allow BCS and, prediction of clinical response. A sequential regimen consisting of four cycles of the anthracyclines, followed by four cycles of Taxotere, achieves improved rates of clinical and pathological response, compared to 4 cycles of anthracycline therapy alone though to date this has not translated to improved survival.

Progressive disease is a rare phenomenon during neoadjuvant chemotherapy but should it occur, a switch should take place either to second line chemotherapy or to surgery. Around 50% of patients will have adequate tumor regression to avoid mastectomy. MRI appears to be the best imaging modality to assess response to neoadjuvant chemotherapy.

Neoadjuvant Endocrine Therapy

A number of large robust randomized trials have proven the benefits of neoadjuvant AI's, particularly letrozole, compared with tamoxifen as first line treatment for large operable tumors in postmenopausal women with Estrogen positive cancers. Letrozole when given for three to four months pre-operatively is superior to tamoxifen in terms of clinical response and rates of BCS, in women who would otherwise require mastectomy. The AI's appear to achieve a much higher response rate than tamoxifen in the subset of patients whose tumors overexpress the HER2 receptor. Prolonged courses increase the numbers of patients who can be treated with BCS.

Neoadjuvant Trastuzumab

In tumors which overexpress HER2, a combination of trastuzumab and chemotherapy achieve superior response rates compared to chemotherapy alone. Pathological complete remission is also increased. In the setting of neoadjuvant treatment of large and locally advanced HER2 positive breast cancers it may soon become standard care.

Follow Up of Patients after Surgery, Risk Factors for Local Recurrence and Survival Outcomes

The risk of local disease recurrence following BCS remains at a fixed rate each year, with rates of less than 1% per year achievable. Following mastectomy it is highest in the first 2 years and decreases with time. Follow up protocols should reflect this. The aim of follow up is to detect local recurrences, new cancers in the treated breast and contralateral disease and, to improve disease free and overall survival through early detection.

Now less than 50% of so called recurrences after BCS are true recurrences and occur at the site of the original breast cancer. Approximately 80% of true recurrences in the conserved breast occur at the site of the original breast cancer. Isolated recurrences can be treated by re-excision or mastectomy but re-excision is associated with a high rate of subsequent local recurrence. Early recurrences are associated with a worse long-term outlook compared to those occurring after 5 years. Those occurring beyond 5 years are likely to represent new primary cancers rather than true recurrences. The remaining "recurrences" in the first 5 years not at the primary tumor site and almost all those occurring beyond 5 years are new primary cancers.

Breast cancer patients are at a greater risk than the general population, of developing a new contralateral cancer (0.6% per year). Annual or biannual mammography to age 80 is advocated but, as a consequence of the degree of scar tissue and distortion caused by BCS, can sometimes be difficult to interpret and to differentiate from local recurrence. MRI can be useful in this setting.

Selected Readings

Al-Ghazal SK, Fallowfield L, Blamey RW (2000) Comparison of psychological aspects and patient satisfaction following breast conserving surgery, simple mastectomy and breast reconstruction. Cancer 36:1938–1943

Allweis TM, Badriyyah Bar ADV, et al. (2003) Current controversies in sentinel lymph node biopsy for breast cancer. Breast 12:163–171

ATAC Trialists Group (2002) Anastrazole alone or in combination with tamoxifen versus tamoxifen alone for adjuvant treatment of postmenopausal women with early breast cancer; first results of the ATAC randomised trial. Lancet 359:2131–2139

Berg WA, Guttierrez L, Ness Avier MS, et al. (2004) Diagnostic accuracy of mammography, clinical examination, US and MR imaging in preoperative assessment of breast cancer. Radiology 233:830–849

Briton LA, Devesa SS (1996) Aetiology and pathogenesis of breast cancer: incidence, demographics and environmental factors. In: Harris JR, Lippman ME, Morrow M, Hellman S (eds) Diseases of the breast. Lippincott-Raven, Philadelphia, pp. 159–168

Dixon JM (2006a) A companion to specialist surgical practice: breast surgery, 3rd edn. Elsevier/W.B. Saunders, London

Dixon JM (2006b) ABC of breast diseases, 3rd edn. BMJ Books/ Blackwell Publishing, London/Oxford

Early Breast Cancer Trialists' Collaborative Group (1996) Favourable and unfavourable effects on long-term survival of radiotherapy for early breast cancer; an overview of the randomised trials. Lancet 348:1189–1196

Early Breast Cancer Trialists' Collaborative Group (1998) Polychemotherapy for early breast cancer: an overview of the randomised trials. Lancet 352:930–942

Early Breast Cancer Trialists' Collaborative Group (2005) Effects of chemotherapy and hormone; therapy for early breast cancer on recurrence and 15 year survival: an overview of the randomised trials. Lancet 365:1687–1717

Singletary SE (2002) Surgical margins in patients with early stage breast cancer treated by breast conserving therapy. Am J Surg 184:383–393

Smith IE, Dowsett M (2003) Aromatase inhibitors in breast cancer. N Eng J Med 348:2431–2442

Veronesi U, Cascinelli N, Mariani L, et al. (2002) Twenty-year follow up of a randomised study comparing breast conserving surgery with radical mastectomy for early breast cancer. N Eng J Med 347:11227–11232

6
Locally Advanced Breast Cancer

Aleksandra Kuciejewska and Ian E. Smith

Pearls and Pitfalls

- Locally advanced breast cancer (LABC) is largely a clinical diagnosis; core biopsy is necessary to characterize the tumor as fully as possible.
- First-line surgery or radiotherapy is usually inappropriate.
- Combined-modality therapy is the standard of care.
- Preoperative chemotherapy or endocrine therapy can downstage initially inoperable cancers to allow surgical resection.
- Mastectomy is the usual surgical choice of surgery; breast conservation is occasionally possible in carefully selected patients.
- Radiotherapy should usually be given after mastectomy, even when response to medical therapy has been good.
- Beware the diagnosis of infection in a young woman with an inflamed breast, without a rapid response to antibiotics.
- Inflammatory breast cancer (IBC) remains a most aggressive subtype. HER-2 analysis is mandatory since there is a high incidence of overexpression here for which treatment with trastuzumab (Herceptin) is likely to be appropriate.

LABC is a heterogeneous and relatively rare form of breast cancer which is either extensive in the breast or in the ipsilateral regional node areas, or both. The tumor is usually large (>5 cm), although size is not an absolute criterion,

K.I. Bland et al. (eds.), *Surgery in Breast Cancer and Melanoma*, DOI 10.1007/978-1-84996-435-7_6,
© Springer-Verlag London Limited 2011

and the definition is based on one or more of the following characteristics:

- Skin or chest wall involvement
- Fixed axillary lymph nodes
- Involvement of ipsilateral internal mammary, supraclavicular or infraclavicular nodes

LABC is usually inoperable, although clinical Stage T3 N0–1 by the American Joint Committee on Cancer system (which implies potential operability) is included in most studies.

In the TNM and stage grouping systems, LABC is defined as:

T0–2 N2 M0 or T3 N1–2 M0 – Stage IIIa
T4 N any M0 or T any N3 M0 – Stage IIIb

IBC is a distinct subtype of LABC associated with a particularly poor prognosis (see below). Neglected or progressive LABC can develop secondary inflammatory features, but should be distinguished from primary IBC as the prognosis differs significantly, and principles of management likewise may differ.

According to the statistics of Cancer Research UK over 40,000 women in the UK are diagnosed with breast cancer each year, but only around 5–10% of these will present with LABC. The incidence is probably higher in developing countries, where there are no screening programs and there is much less social emphasis on breast self-awareness.

Clinical Presentation

The diagnosis of LABC is mainly made on clinical criteria. Patients present with a large breast mass with nodal, skin, or chest wall involvement. Historically, the criteria for a diagnosis of LABC were defined in a classic study by Haagenson and Stout (1943) who reviewed the records of over 1,000 patients treated with radical mastectomy over a 30-year period and identified clinical features associated with >50% risk of local recurrence and virtually no 5-year survivors. These criteria are summarized in Table 6.1. Medical photographs are a useful tool in monitoring progression of the disease and response to treatment (Fig. 6.1).

TABLE 6.1.   Criteria of inoperability (From Haagensen and Stout, 1943).

Extensive skin edema > 1/3 of the breast

Satellite skin nodules

Inflammatory carcinoma

Supraclavicular and parasternal node involvement

Arm edema

Distant metastases

Any two or more of the following: skin edema < 1/3 of the breast, skin ulceration, tumor fixation to chest wall, axillary nodes > 2.5 cm, fixed axillary nodes

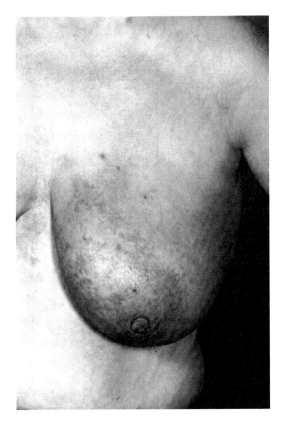

FIGURE 6.1.   Inflammatory breast cancer (IBC).

A full clinical and staging assessment is necessary to exclude distant metastases.

Imaging

Mammography and/or ultrasound may be used as for early breast cancer although the diagnosis is usually obvious clinically. In extreme cases of LABC (bleeding or fungating breast mass), a mammogram may not be appropriate. Ultrasound is a valuable method of documenting tumor size, extension, and regional node involvement before starting treatment. It is also a good method of assessing response to systemic treatment. Other staging investigations including computed tomography (CT) scans of the thorax and abdomen (or chest x-ray and liver ultrasound) along with isotopic bone scan are necessary to exclude distant metastases.

Pathology

The diagnosis is established with fine needle aspiration (FNA) and/or core biopsy. Core biopsy allows full characterization of the tumor including Grade (although this can sometimes be difficult on a core biopsy alone), estrogen receptor (ER) and progesterone (PgR) status, HER-2 status, and lymphovascular invasion. FNA can also be useful in assessing lymph node involvement.

Treatment

Historically, LABC was treated with mastectomy, where technically possible, or with high-dose radiotherapy where surgery was not an option. This approach was associated with a high risk of both local and distant disease recurrence and was almost never curative. The modern approach is to use medical treatment first (chemotherapy, endocrine therapy, or both) to downstage the primary tumor prior to local treatment, and to control micro-metastatic spread (Fig. 6.2).

First reports on the use of induction chemotherapy were published in the 1970s. Over the years, trials have confirmed that combined-modality treatment offers the best outcomes. A multidisciplinary approach is currently the standard treatment of both LABC and IBC. The specialists involved (medical

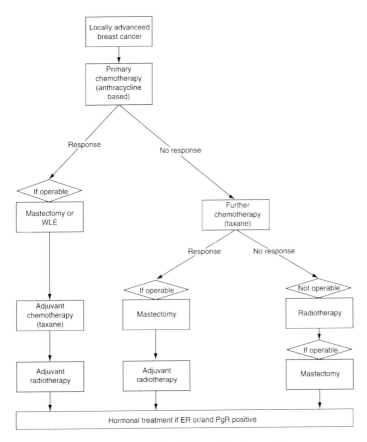

FIGURE 6.2. Treatment algorithm for locally advanced breast cancer.

oncologist, surgeon, and radiotherapist) should review all the available data, and decide collectively on the best combined-modality therapy. Treatment options include systemic treatment (chemotherapy and endocrine therapy) in both the neoadjuvant and adjuvant settings, whereas locoregional treatment involves both surgery and radiotherapy. The literature does not offer extensive level I evidence for treatment of LABC and the majority of recommendations are extrapolated from larger and more recent trials in early breast cancer.

Chemotherapy

Chemotherapy prior to locoregional treatment is a standard management of most patients with LABC. In older patients with ER-positive disease, endocrine primary therapy may be more appropriate (see below).

The main aims of using primary systemic treatment are to:

- Downstage the disease (effect on both tumor and involved nodes) to achieve operability or failing this, to reduce tumor volume prior to radiotherapy
- Use the tumor as an in vivo measure of chemosensitivity
- Achieve early treatment of potential micrometastases

Clinical measurements after each cycle are important to assess response to treatment and in some cases serial ultrasound measurements are also helpful.

Chemotherapy Options

Anthracycline-based schedules are the mainstay of treatment and several different schedules are available including AC (Adriamycin, cyclophosphamide), FAC (5FU), and FEC (epirubicin). It is our practice to continue treatment for six cycles providing good response is achieved, prior to local regional therapy. Taxanes are increasingly used following anthracyclines either as standard or if there is no response after 2–3 cycles of anthracyclines.

Endocrine Therapy

For older women with hormone receptor-positive disease, endocrine therapy may be more appropriate than chemotherapy as initial treatment. The main aim of treatment, as with chemotherapy, is to downstage the tumor to render it operable or to allow conservative surgery instead of mastectomy.

For many years, tamoxifen was the treatment of choice, but recent trials in patients with large operable breast cancers have demonstrated that both letrozole and anastrozole are superior to tamoxifen in terms of downstaging to avoid mastectomy. Response rates of around 50% are achieved. By extrapolation, this approach would also seem appropriate for selected patients with LABC.

A key issue, not yet resolved, concerns the selection of patients for endocrine therapy versus chemotherapy. One small trial has so far compared directly neoadjuvant chemotherapy (Adriamycin and paclitaxel) with an aromatase inhibitor (exemestane or anastrozole). Results have only been reported to date in abstract form, but have shown an overall response rate of 76% for chemotherapy versus 80% for exemestane and 91% for anastrozole. Breast-conserving surgery was achieved more frequently with aromatase inhibitors than with chemotherapy. This important question needs to be addressed in larger trials.

Adjuvant endocrine therapy after locoregional therapy is appropriate for all patients with hormone receptor-positive disease irrespective of preoperative treatment.

Surgery

Surgery is feasible after preoperative chemotherapy in the majority of patients, and indeed breast conservation is sometimes achievable. Breast-conserving surgery should only be performed on carefully selected patients who achieve excellent response with neoadjuvant chemotherapy and when achievement of clear pathological margins is feasible.

A large cohort study of patients with LABC treated with neoadjuvant chemotherapy and breast-conserving surgery implemented strict exclusion criteria (assessed after completion of chemotherapy): residual tumor larger than 5 cm, residual skin edema, direct skin involvement, chest wall fixation, diffuse microcalcifications, multicentric disease, or medical contraindications for the use of radiotherapy. This study reported locoregional relapse rates of 10% in Stage IIIa and 15% in Stage IIIb disease. As expected, the tumor size and extent of nodal involvement influenced markedly the rate of the recurrence (T1–2 7% vs. T3–4 14%; N0–1 7% vs. N2–3 16%).

Providing there are no medical contraindications it is also important to perform adequate axillary node dissection, since the risk of persisting nodal involvement is high.

Radiotherapy

Radiotherapy plays an important role in locoregional treatment of LABC and is indicated usually after surgery, or alone when the primary tumor remains inoperable after neoadjuvant medical therapy. The main aim of postoperative radiotherapy is to reduce the risk of local recurrence following surgery, or to achieve local control where the primary tumor is inoperable.

Our policy is to deliver tangential-field radiotherapy to the chest wall and supraclavicular fossa (provided that four or more axillary nodes were involved) with a boost to the original tumor bed following conservative surgery in patients of 50 years old and younger. Irradiation of axillary nodes will be considered if extracapsular spread was seen on the pathology sample or if no axillary surgery was performed. A standard dose of radiation is 50 Gy in 25 fractions or equivalent with the boost dose of 16 Gy in eight fractions, using electron energy. When irradiating IBC, bolus is applied to the skin usually for most of the time of radiotherapy, depending on skin tolerance.

In inoperable tumors whole breast radiotherapy is recommended in the dose of 50 Gy in 25 fractions with the boost dose of 16 Gy.

Trastuzumab (Herceptin)

HER-2/neu (also known as c-erbB-2) is a transmembrane growth factor from the epidermal growth factor (EGFR) family of tyrosine kinases. Significant overexpression of HER-2 occurs in approximately 20% of all breast cancers and HER-2 positivity is linked with a more aggressive course of disease and worse prognosis.

The humanized monoclonal antibody against HER-2 protein, trastuzumab (Herceptin), improves survival when given with chemotherapy in the treatment of patients with metastatic, HER-2-positive breast cancer. Recently published trials have shown that, when used in early breast cancer after adjuvant chemotherapy, or concomitantly with taxane adjuvant chemotherapy, trastuzumab decreases the early risk of recurrence by around 50%.

In a small randomized neoadjuvant trial, trastuzumab with chemotherapy improved very significantly the clinical and pathological remission rates compared with chemotherapy alone.

Putting these results together, it is our view that all LABCs should be tested for HER-2 protein overexpression by immunohistochemistry (IHC) or gene amplification using fluorescence in situ hybridization (FISH), and if chemotherapy is indicated and the tumor is HER-2-positive, trastuzumab should be used in addition.

Prognosis and Prognostic Factors

Features of LABC which can help to establish prognosis are listed in Table 6.2. Since the use of combined-modality treatment, the prognosis of LABC has improved markedly. Current data suggest that for Stage IIIa the 10-year survival

TABLE 6.2. Prognostic factors of locally advanced breast cancer (LABC).

Size
Grade
Number of nodes involved
Stage
Hormone receptor status
Menopausal status if ER/PgR-positive, as the estrogen levels are naturally much lower HER-2 status
Response to primary chemotherapy or endocrine therapy

is over 50%, while for Stage IIIb (excluding IBC), the survival figures remain low at 30%.

Inflammatory Breast Cancer

IBC is an aggressive but uncommon clinical subtype of LABC, with an overall incidence of 1–6% of all invasive breast cancers. The incidence has doubled approximately in the last 20 years. IBC is defined on the basis of clinical findings and pathological features.

Clinical findings include:

- Rapidly progressing erythema
- Increased temperature of effected skin
- Edema of the breast, often with breast enlargement
- Peau d'orange and ridging
- Diffuse firmness on palpation
- A well-defined mass often not palpable and/or not found on mammogram
- Dermal lymphatic invasion is present in most patients, but this is not a determinant of diagnosis

Significant clinical findings of IBC can be associated with minimal radiological abnormalities and a radiologically defined mass may not be present. Instead imaging can show nonspecific signs such as a generalized increase in breast tissue density or thickening of the skin, as well as large areas of calcification or parenchymal distortion.

There are several features of IBC that make it phenotypically distinct and could explain partially its aggressive nature and these are listed in Table 6.3. These biological characteristics of IBC tumors may provide molecular targets for new treatments.

Historically, IBC was treated with either mastectomy or radiation, but both treatments resulted in very high rates of local and distant recurrence with few survivors beyond 5 years. Today, IBC should be treated initially with chemotherapy as part of a combined-modality approach, with up to 50% patients surviving for 5 years.

The schedules of primary chemotherapy are similar to those for the treatment of other forms of LABC. The use of taxanes after anthracycline-based chemotherapy is becoming more common. Depending on the response to chemotherapy, patients proceed either to surgery (usually mastectomy if the disease has become resectable) followed by radiotherapy, or to radiotherapy alone if surgery is not possible.

Given the aggressive clinical course of IBC and high rate of HER-2/neu overexpression, combining targeted agents with chemotherapy in the neoadjuvant setting may prove beneficial, especially as the trastuzumab/chemotherapy combination has shown already excellent results in adjuvant and

TABLE 6.3. Phenotypical features of inflammatory breast cancer (IBC).

HER-2/neu overexpression is higher (around 50%) than in noninflammatory breast cancers

Frequently negative ER receptor status

High mitotic index

More pronounced angiogenesis

High rate of p53 overexpression

Increased MUC1 staining and E-cadherin

metastatic settings. In a preliminary study of women with HER-2-positive LABC, trastuzumab was employed with docetaxel in the neoadjuvant setting and all nine patients with IBC responded to treatment.

Lapatinib, a reversible dual inhibitor of ErbB1 and ErbB2 tyrosine kinases, is currently under investigation. Results of a Phase I trial demonstrated clinical activity of lapatinib in heavily pretreated patients with metastatic IBC whose tumors overexpressed erbB2 and erbB1 and who had progressed despite prior trastuzumab-containing regimens. Further trials are now investigating the use of lapatinib as a part of neoadjuvant treatment for IBC on its own and in conjunction with taxane chemotherapy.

Finally, it should be noted that some IBCs are hormone receptor-positive, and in older patients or those otherwise unfit for chemotherapy, a trial of endocrine therapy is warranted.

Selected Readings

Burris HA, Hurwitz HI, Dees EC, et al. (2005) Phase I safety, pharmacokinetics, and clinical activity study of lapatinib (GW572016), a reversible dual inhibitor of epidermal growth factor receptor tyrosine kinases, in heavily pretreated patients with metastatic carcinomas. J Clin Oncol 23:5305–5315

Buzdar AU, Ibrahim NK, Francis D, et al. (2005) Significantly higher pathologic complete remission rate after neoadjuvant therapy with Trastuzumab, Paclitaxel, and Epirubicin chemotherapy: results of a randomised trial in human epidermal growth factor receptor 2-positive operable breast cancer. J Clin Oncol 23:3676–3685

Chen AM, Meric-Bernstam F, Hunt KK, et al. (2004) Breast conservation after neoadjuvant chemotherapy: the M.D. Anderson Cancer Center experience. J Clin Oncol 22:2303–2312

Eiermann W, Paepke S, Appfelstaedt J, et al. (2001) Pre-operative treatment of postmenopausal breast cancer patients with letrozole: a randomised double-blind multi-center study. Ann Oncol 12:1527–1532

Low JA, Berman AW, Steinberg SM, et al. (2004) Long-term follow-up for locally advanced and inflammatory breast cancer patients treated with multimodality therapy. J Clin Oncol 22:4067–4074

Piccart-Gebhart MJ, Procter M, Leyland-Jones B (2005) Trastuzumab after adjuvant chemotherapy in HER2positive breast cancer. N Engl J Med 353:1659–1671

Romond EH, Perez EA, Bryant J, et al. (2005) Trastuzumab plus adjuvant chemotherapy for operable HER2-positive breast cancer. N Engl J Med 353:1673–1684

Semiglasov VV, Semiglasov VG, Ivanoff EK, et al. (2004) Preoperative hormonal therapy vs. chemotherapy in post menopausal, ER positive breast cancer patients. Eur J Cancer 371

Shenkier T, Weir L, Levine M, et al. (2004) Clinical practice guidelines for the care and treatment of breast cancer:15. Treatment for women with stage III or locally advanced breast cancer. CMAJ 170:983–984

Smith IE, Dowsett M, Ebbs SR, et al. (2005) Neoadjuvant treatment of postmenopausal breast cancer either anastrazole, tamoxifen, or both in combination: the immediate Anastrazole, Tamoxifen, or combined with Tamoxifen (IMPACT) multicenter double-blind randomised trial. J Clin Oncol 23:5108–5116

Toonkel LM, Fix I, Jackobson LH, et al. (1986) Locally advanced breast carcinoma: results with combined regional therapy. Int J Radiat Oncol Biol Phys 12:1583–1587

Van der Hage JA, Van de Velde CJH, Julien JP, et al. (2001) Preoperative chemotherapy in primary operable breast cancer: results from the European Organisation for Research and Treatment of Cancer Trial 10902. J Clin Oncol 19:4224–4237

Van Pelt AE, Mohsin S, Elledge RM, et al. (2003) Neoadjuvant trastuzumab and docetaxel in breast cancer: preliminary results. Clin Breast Cancer 4:348–353

Veronesi U, Bonadonna G, Zurrida S, et al. (1995) Conservation surgery after primary chemotherapy in large carcinomas of the breast. Ann Surg 222:612–618

7
Metastatic Carcinomas of the Breast

Jhanelle Gray and Pamela N. Munster

Pearls and Pitfalls

- Metastatic breast cancer remains incurable; however, appropriately targeted therapy will prolong survival.
- The assessment of estrogen, progesterone, and HER2/*neu* receptor expression status are crucial for optimal therapy.
- Patients whose tumors overexpress HER2/*neu* should be treated with trastuzumab either alone or in combination with chemotherapy.
- Premenopausal women with hormone-receptor positive metastatic breast cancer should be considered for tamoxifen with or without oophorectomy or Luteinizing-Hormone-Releasing Hormone (LHRH) agonist for combined hormonal blockade.
- Postmenopausal women with hormone-receptor positive metastatic breast cancer should be treated with tamoxifen or an aromatase inhibitor.
- Patients with hormone-receptor positive tumors in visceral crisis or with impending spinal cord compression will likely require chemotherapy initially.
- The continued participation in clinical trials evaluating novel agents is an important contribution in the attempt to cure, prolong life, and alleviate symptoms.

K.I. Bland et al. (eds.), *Surgery in Breast Cancer and Melanoma*, DOI 10.1007/978-1-84996-435-7_7,
© Springer-Verlag London Limited 2011

Introduction

Breast cancer is the most common type of cancer in women. While the incidence of breast cancer has continued to rise, the mortality has now begun to decrease in part due to earlier detection and improved therapeutic modalities. The majority of women present after the age of 50. Bone, brain, liver, and lung are the major sites of metastatic involvement. Metastatic breast cancer remains incurable. However, the successful recognition of pathways responsible for the development and progression of breast cancer and the introduction of many novel cytotoxic agents, as well as targeted therapies, has not only prolonged the survival of patients, but also improved their quality of life.

Clinical Presentation

There is no typical presentation for patients with metastatic breast cancer. Patients may have asymptomatic disease with laboratory abnormalities, such as a rise in tumor markers, or present with a symptom due to a specific metastatic lesion. Some patients can present with more vague symptoms such as fatigue, malaise, and weight loss. In others, metastatic disease is found during a routine clinical exam or during scheduled or incidental radiological tests. Despite a concerted effort for early detection, some patients still present with primary metastatic disease.

Diagnosis

Once metastatic disease is suspected, at least one site should be biopsied to obtain pathological confirmation of metastatic involvement and to reassess the estrogen receptor (ER), progesterone receptor (PR), and HER2/*neu* status of the metastatic tumors which often differ from the initial tumor. This information may broaden or narrow the therapeutic options for the patients. In patients with bone metastases, biopsies may be more challenging. Single metastatic sites should always be biopsied, particularly isolated lung metastases. In patients with a smoking history, approximately 50% of these lesions may represent lung cancer, which may be curable with appropriate surgical resection. A complete white blood cell count and routine blood chemistry should be performed. These will reflect upon the bone marrow reserve and organ function, which will assess any functional compromise and the need for therapy modification. Patients should undergo staging studies not only to determine the extent of the metastatic involvement, but also to be able to assess the response to therapy. These include a contrast-enhanced CT scan of the chest and abdomen and, depending on symptoms, also of the pelvis. Given the frequent involvement of sclerotic and lytic bone lesions, a bone scan should be included. While FDG-PET scans have been shown to have a role in several solid tumor malignancies, the use of FDG-PET scans in breast cancer is controversial due to limited predictability. In addition, PET-CT scans may not allow the appropriate sizing of tumor lesions. A MRI of the brain should be considered due to the incidence of asymptomatic brain metastasis (10–15%). Tumor markers such as carcinoembryonic antigen (CEA) and CA 15-3 may be considered an adjunct to follow therapy response; however, the mere elevation of such tumor markers should not determine the diagnosis of metastatic disease or prompt the initiation of cytotoxic therapy.

Therapeutic Decisions

Therapy for ER/PR Positive Tumors

In 1896 Beatson observed a regression of breast tumors in women undergoing an oophorectomy. This was the beginning of a long line of successful discoveries in terms of hormonal manipulations as a means of treatment for hormone-sensitive breast cancer. This modality, however, was only useful for premenopausal women. Since the majority of women are diagnosed with metastatic breast cancer beyond the age of 50, only a limited number of patients benefited. About 50 years later, it was demonstrated that resection of the adrenal glands also led to regression; however, this approach was more effective in post-menopausal women. The estrogen withdrawal by a surgical approach has been largely replaced by a chemical approach, either by the modulation or down-regulation of the estrogen receptor by selective estrogen-receptor modulators (SERMs) by or selective estrogen-receptor down-regulators (SERDs) by and agents blocking the conversion of estrogen from its precursors by aromatase inhibitors (AIs). Other modalities such as the use of a synthetic progesterone like megestrol acetate (Megace), androgens, or even the use of high doses of estrogen are effective. However, due to their undesirable side effects, they are less commonly used or are used at a later stage.

Premenopausal Women

The main treatment option for pre-menopausal women with estrogen-receptor or progesterone-receptor positive tumors is tamoxifen (Fig. 7.1). Tamoxifen (Nolvadex) is an oral SERM. SERMs act by competing with estrogen for the estrogen receptor; due to differential regulation of co-activators and co-repressors, the effects of SERMs are tissue-specific and may be pro-estrogenic in some tissues and anti-estrogenic in others which explains the observed adverse effects. Tamoxifen use has demonstrated response rates ranging from 16–56%, duration of responses lasting 12–18 months, and a decrease in breast cancer-related mortality. Tamoxifen side effects include: hot flashes, deep venous thrombosis, pulmonary emboli, stroke, and endometrial cancer, but may also have protective effects on the bones. Due to the pro-thrombotic effects of tamoxifen, smoking cessation is strongly encouraged and patients should be instructed to avoid prolonged inactivity, particularly on airplanes.

Many patients will develop resistance to the drug. Tamoxifen should be discontinued upon evidence of progressive disease. If use is continued, it has been demonstrated that tamoxifen

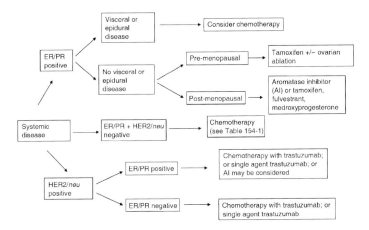

FIGURE 7.1. Metastatic breast cancer treatment.

can exert agonist properties at its site of action, leading to tumor progression. In addition, following cessation of tamoxifen at the time of progressive disease, tumor regression has been seen in some patients.

In pre-menopausal women, the ovaries are responsible for the majority of the estrogen released into circulation. Bilateral oophorectomies are an acceptable method in this patient population for achieving estrogen suppression. Ovarian ablation can also be accomplished by ovarian radiation or the use of Luteinizing-Hormone-Releasing Hormone agonist (LHRH-agonist), which is commonly given as a one- or three-monthly injection. A combined analysis of several smaller studies has shown that the use of tamoxifen in conjunction with ovarian ablation has resulted in improved disease-free and overall survival compared to either tamoxifen or ovarian ablation alone.

Hormonal Interventions in Post-Menopausal Women

Menopause is defined as the cessation of menstrual cycles for 6–12 months. However, this definition should be used with caution in younger women who have been treated with chemotherapy. Chemotherapy-induced amenorrhea may be reversible up to several months and even years after completion of chemotherapy. This should be particularly considered when treating patients with agents that are only effective in a low-estrogenic environment, such as the AIs.

For many years, tamoxifen has been the treatment of choice in post-menopausal women with ER and/or PR positive breast cancer. This has been challenged with the introduction of the selective AIs. After cessation of ovarian function, the adrenal glands are the major source of endogenous estrogen. The surgical removal of the adrenal glands is an effective modality; however, the impact on the gluco- and mineralo-corticosteroid hormones induced by this approach has significant side effects. The introduction of the oral agent aminoglutethimide (which had not been approved for this purpose by the Food and Drug Administration at the time of publication) was one of the first successful non-surgical methods of blocking the production of estrogen. However, aminoglutethimide is non-selective and blocks an early step in the generation of steroid, the conversion of cholesterol to delta-5-pregnenolone, thereby blocking all adrenal steroids, including glucocorticoids, mineralocorticoids, and estrogen. Aminoglutethimide has now been replaced by more selective AIs which block the conversion of androgenic precursors to estrogens (androstenedione to estradiol and testosterone to estrone). Unlike the surgical approach, the AIs also block estrogen conversion in other sites including the breast, adipose tissue, liver, muscles, and brain. The most commonly used AIs for metastatic disease are the reversible, non-steroidal AIs: anastrazole (Arimidex) and letrozole (Femara); and the irreversible steroidal AI: exemestane (Aromasin). All three have been compared to tamoxifen in large, randomized phase III trials. In most studies, the AIs were found to improve the response rate, the disease-free survival, and/or the time to disease progression. However, none of the studies suggested an overall survival benefit for AIs versus tamoxifen when given as first-line therapy (Fig. 7.1 and Table 7.1).

TABLE 7.1. Aromatase inhibitors versus tamoxifen in MBC.

Bonnetorre et al., 2000	Anastrazole vs. Tamoxifen	668	32.9% vs. 32.6% NS	8.2 vs. 8.3 months NS
Nabholtz et al., 2000	Anastrazole vs. Tamoxifen	353	21% vs. 17% NS	11.1 vs. 5.6 months P: 0.005
Mouridsen et al., 2001	Letrozole vs. Tamoxifen	907	30% vs. 20% P = 0.0006	10.25 vs. 6.5 months P < 0.001
Paridaens et al., 2004	Exemestane vs. Tamoxifen	382	44% vs. 29% NA	10.9 vs. 6.7 months NA

NS = not significant; NA = not available.

The use of sequential AIs (e.g. a non-steroidal AI followed by a steroid AI upon progression of disease or vice versa) should also be considered as this approach has been shown to be beneficial. The main side effects of AIs are bone loss, fractures, muscle-skeletal effects (such as stiffness and joint pain), gastrointestinal adverse events, and vaginal dryness. Questionable adverse effects on the lipids are currently being studied. Hot flashes are similar to those seen with tamoxifen in some, but not all studies comparing an AI with tamoxifen and may be AI-specific. While thromboembolic events occur, they are less common than those seen with tamoxifen. Neither endometrial hyperplasia nor endometrial cancers have been reported in association with the use of AIs. While the AIs differ in structure and pharmacological profile, it is not yet established whether this will translate into clinical superiority of any of the agents.

Other SERMs and Antiestrogens

Toremifene (Fareston) is an oral SERM that has been FDA approved for use in post-menopausal women. Three large phase III trials have compared toremifene to tamoxifen in post-menopausal women with hormone-receptor positive or unknown receptor status advanced-stage breast cancer, and no differences between response rate, time to progression, and overall survival were found. Due to the potential for cross-resistance to tamoxifen, it is rarely used as second-line therapy in tamoxifen failures.

Another approach to patients who progress on anti-hormonal therapy is the pure anti-estrogen (or SERD), fulvestrant (Faslodex). It is administered by a monthly intramuscular injection and has comparable response rates and time to progression as AIs. EM 800 is another "pure" anti-estrogen. This oral drug is being evaluated in a phase III clinical trial. Other potential therapies for patients with metastatic hormone-receptor positive breast cancer include: antiprogestins, antiandrogens and androgens, estrogens, glucocorticoids, and somatostatins.

Ongoing Clinical Trials and Future Directions

Clinical trials are ongoing to investigate and discover novel agents or new combinations that will increase overall survival for hormone-positive metastatic breast cancer. These include trials evaluating AIs combined with oral EGFR inhibitors or other novel agents, including sorafenib (Nexavar), which inhibits RAS oncogene, VEGF, and PDGF pathways, and SCH66336 (Lonafarnib), which inhibits farnesyltransferase. A more complete list can be found at www.clinicaltrials.gov.

HER2/neu

HER2/neu (erbB-2), human epidermal growth factor, is a transmembrane tyrosine kinase receptor expressed in breast cancer cells. While HER2/neu does not have a known ligand, there is cross-talk between other receptors in the erbB family, including HER1 (EGFR), HER3, and HER4. HER2/neu is believed to be activated by hetero-dimerization with these receptors and by autophosphorylation due to homo-dimerization with itself.

This leads to downstream intracellular signaling which is important for cell proliferation.

HER2/*neu* is overexpressed in about 20–30% of breast cancers. Measurement of overexpression is done by either protein overexpression using immunohistochemistry (IHC) and quantified as 0, 1+, 2+, or 3+; or by gene amplification as defined by an increase in the expression of HER2/*neu* copies compared to chromosome 17 by fluorescent in situ hybridization (FISH). A ratio greater than 2.2 is considered amplified. Detection by FISH has been shown to be more predictive of response and should now be considered in all patients, particularly those with 2+ protein overexpression. Many of these patients will not demonstrate a gene amplification by FISH.

Agents Targeting HER2/neu

The development of the humanized, monoclonal antibody, trastuzumab (Herceptin), has been a significant milestone in the treatment of HER2/*neu* overexpressing breast cancer (Fig. 7.1). Trastuzumab binds to the extracellular domain of the receptor. Trastuzumab is delivered intravenously with an initial bolus followed by weekly or every 3 week administration. As monotherapy, response rates of 26% for first line therapy and 15% for second or third line therapy have been demonstrated in patients who have protein overexpression of 2+ or 3+ by IHC. The response rates were 35%, when only patients with 3+ overexpression were analyzed.

Care must be taken when administering trastuzumab. Approximately 2–5% of patients will develop cardiac dysfunction (grade 3 and 4), even when used as a single agent. Careful monitoring of the ejection fraction is advisable during therapy.

Trastuzumab and Chemotherapy

To date, numerous clinical trials have been performed to evaluate the use of trastuzumab in combination with chemotherapy agents (Table 7.2). In the pivotal phase III trial, the response rates for anthracycline-based therapy plus trastuzumab were 50% versus 23% for anthracyclines alone, with a time to progression of 7.4 versus 4.6 months, and an overall survival of 25.1 versus 20.3 months. Despite these promising results, these two medications should not be combined due to excessive cardiac toxicity. A combination of trastuzumab with a taxane, either docetaxel and paclitaxel, nearly doubled the response rates and time to progression compared to chemotherapy alone, while the overall survival increased by 3.7–5.7 months without excessive cardiac events. The use of triple therapy with paclitaxel and trastuzumab plus carboplatin (which had not been approved for this purpose by the Food and Drug Administration at the time of publication) yielded response rates of 52%, while vinorelbine (which also had not been approved for this purpose by the Food and Drug Administration at the time of publication) and trastuzumab had response rates of up to 75%. For extensively treated patients, response rates for trastuzumab in combination with other cytotoxic agents, such as capecitabine, gemcitabine, and liposomal doxorubicin (which also had not been approved for this purpose by the Food and Drug Administration at the time of publication), were 53%, 37%, and 58%, respectively. These serve as further therapeutic options for this patient population.

Although no randomized studies have been performed to specifically answer the question, many physicians and patients hesitate to discontinue trastuzumab upon progression of disease following one regimen.

New Agents

Several other agents targeting HER2/*neu* are being explored and are at various stages of clinical development. These include lapatinib, HKI-272, and others. Unlike the monoclonal antibody trastuzumab, lapatinib (Tykerb) and HKI-272 (which had not been approved for this purpose by the Food and Drug Administration at the time of publication) are oral

TABLE 7.2. Combination regimens that have shown a survival benefit over a single agent.

Source	Regimen	N	RR	TTP or PFSa	Median survival
O'Shaughnessy et al., 2002	Docetaxel 75 mg/m^2 plus Capecitabine 1,250 mg/m^2 bid vs. Docetaxel 100 mm/m^2	511	42% vs. 30% P: 0.006	6.1 vs. 4.2 months P: 0.0001	14.5 vs. 11.5 months P: 0.0126
Albain et al., 2004	Paclitaxel plus Gemcitabine vs. Paclitaxel	529	40.8% vs. 22.10% P < 0.0001	5.2 vs. 2.9 months P < 0.0001	18.5 vs. 15.8 months
Slamon et al., 2001	Chemotherapy^b plus trastuzumab vs. chemotherapy alone	496	50% vs. 32% P < 0.001	7.4 vs. 4.6 months P < 0.001	25.1 vs. 20.3 months P = 0.008
Marty et al., 2005	Docetaxel plus Trastuzumab vs. Docetaxel alone	186	61% vs.34% P = 0.0002	11.7 vs. 6.1 months P = 0.0001	31.2 vs. 22.7 months P = 0.0325
Robert et al., 2006	Trastuzumab, Paclitaxel, and Carboplatin vs. Trastuzumab and Paclitaxel	196	52% vs. 36% P = 0.04	10.7 vs. 7.1 months P = 0.03	35.7 vs. 32.2 months NS

NA = not available.

aTTP = time to progression; PFS = progression free survival.

bChemotherapy = Adriamycin and Cyclophosphamide or Paclitaxel. Adriamycin should not be combined with Trastuzumab due to the development of congestive heart failure.

kinase inhibitors that target not only HER2/*neu*, but also the erbB1 receptor. In the December 2006 publication of the New England Journal of Medicine (NEJM), the data from a phase III trial evaluating the use of lapatinib plus capecitabine versus capecitabine alone was published by Geyer et al. The study included individuals with HER2/*neu* positive advanced or metastatic breast cancer who had been previously treated. The combination of the two agents was associated with an improved progression-free survival. Very few patients were found to have adverse effects on the heart, but the effects were reversible in all patients.

Tumors with HER2/neu and Estrogen Overexpression

There is conflicting data on the use of hormonal therapy combined with trastuzumab in patients with HER2/*neu* and ER positive metastatic breast cancer. Some of the evidence suggests that overexpression of HER2/*neu* may cause resistance to hormonal therapy in patients that are ER positive. At this point there is no clear data advocating the combined use of trastuzumab and anti-hormonal therapy in patients with metastatic breast cancer. While tamoxifen is believed to be less effective in patients with HER2/*neu* overexpression, the AIs have shown efficacy and should be considered. A phase IV clinical trial is currently ongoing to evaluate the combination of letrozole and trastuzumab.

Further clinical trials are evaluating the use of trastuzumab in combination with other inhibitors of the erBb-kinase family, as well as the addition of lapatinib.

ER/PR Negative and HER2/neu Negative Tumors

Patients who have metastatic breast cancer and are ER/PR negative and HER2/*neu* negative will derive most of their benefit from cytotoxic therapy (Fig. 7.1). Response rates can be as high as 50–70%. Several classes of cytotoxic agents have demonstrated activity in patients with metastatic breast cancer and have been tested either alone or in combination with other drugs (Tables 7.2 and 7.3).

Combination Versus Single Agent

Many cytotoxic agents have been used as monotherapy for treatment of metastatic breast cancer including anthracyclines, taxanes, and alkylating agents (Table 7.3). Response rates for these agents range from 10–60%. Many of the trials suggest an increase in the response rate and an increase in the time to tumor progression, but few trials have shown a survival benefit when using multiple agents compared to a single agent (Table 7.2). A survival benefit was demonstrated when combining docetaxel with capecitabine compared to docetaxel alone, and gemcitabine in combination with paclitaxel compared to paclitaxel alone. However, in these trials, the effects of the combination regimen have been compared to a single agent and have not evaluated the use of both drugs in sequence. A pivotal trial compared the survival of patients treated with a combination of Adriamycin and paclitaxel to those treated with each drug alone. Upon progression, patients treated with a single agent were allowed to cross over to another agent. While the combination arm showed an improved response rate and time to progression, there was no difference in survival and the combination was associated with more toxicity.

While combination regimens should be used with caution, they may prove beneficial in a patient with rapidly progressing visceral metastases. The debate whether to use combination agents versus a single agent is based on the principle of utilizing agents with differing mechanisms of actions to minimize resistance, increase tumor killing, and eradicate all tumor cells. This concept has been successfully implemented in cancers such as Hodgkin's disease and testicular cancer, even in patients with widely metastatic disease. While this concept has been tested in breast cancer, several studies have shown that even the use of high dose therapy with stem cell

TABLE 7.3. Single agents that have demonstrated activity in breast cancer.

Class	Generic examples	Common side effects	Rare, severe side effects
Anthracyclines	Doxorubicin Epirubicin Liposomal Doxorubicin[a]	Nausea, vomiting, alopecia, myelosuppression	Pericarditis-myocarditis syndrome, Cardio-myopathy (>400 mg/m² for Doxorubicin; > 750 mg/m² for Epirubicin), secondary acute myelogenous leukemia, diarrhea, anal fissures
Alkylating agents	Cyclophosphamide	Nausea, vomiting, alopecia, myelosuppression	Hemorrhagic cystitis (20%), elevated LFT's, hepatitis, jaundice, interstitial, pulmonary fibrosis, CHF (at doses of 120–170 mg/kg over days)
Antimetabolites	Methotrexate	Myelosuppression, mucositis, skin erythema, pruritus, photosensitivity, increased LFT's	Alopecia, renal tubular damage, encephalopathy (w/ multiple intracranial doses), fetal loss or congenital malformations in 1st trimester, allergic rxn
Fluoropyrimidines	5-fluorouracil, Capecitabine	Mucositis, diarrhea, nausea, vomiting, stomatitis, dysphagia, myelosuppression, alopecia, hand-and-foot syndrome, fatigue	MI (2%), conjunctivitis, lacrimation, blepharites, photophobia, somnolence and cerebellar ataxia (1%), headache, paresthesia

Taxanes	Paclitaxel Docetaxel ABI 007	Peripheral neuropathy, myelosuppression, nausea, vomiting, myalgias, mild LFT elevation, mucositis, alopecia, edema	Seizures, hypertension, bradycardia, arrhythmias, hypersensitivity reactions, skin toxicity
Anti-metabolites	Gemcitabine[a]	Myelosuppression, nausea, vomiting, diarrhea, stomatitis, mild proteinuria and hematuria, transient elevated LFT's, rash, alopecia, fever, edema	Myelosuppression, pulmonary toxicity
Vinca alkaloids	Vinorelbine[a]	Myelosuppression, peripheral neuropathy, constipation, nausea, vomiting, diarrhea, stomatitis, alopecia	Myelosuppression, myalgias, peritumoral pain, paralytic ileus, allergic rxn, elevated LFT's, SIADH, fatigue, hemorrhagic cystitis
Platinums	Carboplatina Cisplatina	Nausea, vomiting, peripheral neuropathy	Renal failure, electrolyte disturbances, tinnitus, myelosuppression, SIADH, elevated LFT's, bradycardia, hyperuricemia, rash

[a]These drugs have not been approved for this purpose by the Food and Drug Administration at the time of publication.

rescue has not led to durable disease eradication. Hence, the major benefits are more likely to stem from the testing of novel agents and their addition to currently used therapies rather than the combination of standard cytotoxic therapy.

Combination of Cytotoxic Agents with Biologic Agents

Bevacizumab is a humanized monoclonal antibody that inhibits all isoforms of the vascular endothelial growth factor (VEGF), a potent pro-angiogenic peptide. Another drug in the same class is PTK787. It is orally administered and strongly inhibits all VEGF receptors.

The results of a large, randomized trial adding bevacizumab to paclitaxel were reported by Miller et al. in the NEJM in 2007. Adding bevacizumab to paclitaxel prolonged progression-free survival from to 5.9 to 11.0 months and increased the response rate from 21.2% to 36.9%. The bevacizumab arm was associated with a higher rate of hypertension, cerebrovascular ischemia, and proteinuria. This agent appears to be promising for use in the treatment of metastatic breast cancer and was approved by the Food and Drug Administration in 2008. Longer follow-up will be needed to determine the benefit of survival with this regimen.

Promising Novel Strategies of Old Drugs

One of the newer agents that have been developed for use in the metastatic setting is ABI 007 (Abraxane). It is a nanoparticle, albumin-bound paclitaxel that is prepared Cremophor-free. This formulation has increased the therapeutic window, decreased the infusion time, and allowed for the omission of steroid pre-medication. The nanoparticle, albumin-bound paclitaxel has been associated with response rates of 33% versus 19% compared to standard paclitaxel. The nanoparticle, albumin-bound paclitaxel was associated with an increase in sensory neuropathy, but less frequent neutropenia.

Exciting Clinical Trials and Future Directions

New drug combinations and single agents are constantly being developed. Many early trials are underway to evaluate novel agents that inhibit or target pathways associated with tumor development or progression. These include inhibitors of the VEGF (vascular endothelial growth factor) or VEGF receptor, the IGF (insulin growth factor) receptor, the PDGF (platelet derived growth factor) receptor, as well as inhibitors of src, notch, aurora kinase, met, wnt, c-kit signaling, and the novel class of histone deacetylase inhibitors. To increase the efficacy of drugs for the treatment of breast cancer, participation in a clinical trial should be considered. More information regarding clinical trials for patients with metastatic breast cancer can be found at www.clinicaltrials.gov.

Other Systemic Therapy

Bone involvement is common in patients with metastatic breast cancer. The use of bisphosphonates, such as zoledronate and pamidronate, should be highly considered in these patients. Randomized trials have shown a decrease in skeletal morbidity. Care must be taken when administering bisphosphonates, as they carry a risk of renal damage leading to renal insufficiency, and more recently have been associated with osteonecrosis of the jaw. For patients with poor dentition, these drugs should be administered with the guidance of an oral surgeon or dentist. Radiation therapy should also be considered for symptomatic patients.

Role of Surgery

In general, the role of surgery is very limited in patients with metastatic breast cancer. A resection of a metastatic lesion may be considered in patients with symptomatic metastases or oligometastatic disease, particularly of the central nervous system. As this represents such a small patient population, there are no randomized trials that have demonstrated survival data. The benefits of surgery and the potential symptom relief should be carefully weighed against the patient's risk of surgery, comorbidities, and the likelihood of rapid development of other metastatic sites requiring a systemic approach. Stereotactic radiosurgery has emerged as an alternative for surgery in patients with brain metastases. A new lesion in the breast in a patient with a prior history of breast cancer is often resected to distinguish a new primary tumor from a recurrence, as it would alter the therapeutic approach. The resection of a chest wall recurrence may be considered to avoid local complications. However, when other organs are involved with metastatic disease, an easily accessible tumor in the chest wall may provide a means to assess treatment response and obtain tissue for correlative studies in conjunction with clinical trials.

Outcomes

Breast cancer is the second leading cause of cancer-related death. In the metastatic setting, some individuals will have an insidious course while others will have a more rapid course to their disease. The characterization of predictive markers and the introduction of targeted agents have greatly improved the survival and quality of life of patients with metastatic breast cancer. The majority of advances have stemmed from the development of targeted therapy, such as the SERMS or aromatase inhibitors, and the introduction of trastuzumab. Still, the majority of patients with metastatic disease will die of their disease and may have debilitating symptoms. Therefore a continued thrive for early detection and more effective and selective therapies are imperative. The ultimate goal is to have patient-specific, accurate, novel therapies that will impact time to cancer recurrence, as well as outcomes.

Selected Readings

Albain KS, Nag S, Calderillo-Ruiz G, et al. (2004) Global phase III study of gemcitabine plus paclitaxel (GT) vs. paclitaxel (T) as frontline therapy for metastatic breast cancer (MBC): First report of overall survival. ASCO Annual Meeting Proceedings (Post-Meeting Edition) J Clin Onc (Supplemental edition):510

Bonneterre J, Thurlimann B, Robertson JF, et al. (2000) Anastrozole versus tamoxifen as first-line therapy for advanced breast cancer in 668 postmenopausal women: results of the Tamoxifen or Arimidex Randomized Group Efficacy and Tolerability study. J Clin Oncol 18:3748–3757

Burstein HJ, Harris LN, Marcom PK, et al. (2003) Trastuzumab and vinorelbine as first-line therapy for HER2-overexpressing metastatic breast cancer: multicenter phase II trial with clinical outcomes, analysis of serum tumor markers as predictive factors, and cardiac surveillance algorithm. J Clin Oncol 21:2889–2895

Cobleigh MA, Vogel CL, Tripathy D, et al. (1999) Multi-national study of the efficacy and safety of humanized anti-HER2 monoclonal antibody in women who have HER2-overexpressing metastatic breast cancer that has progressed after chemotherapy for metastatic disease. J Clin Oncol 17:2639–2648

Gershanovich M, Garin A, Baltina D, et al. (1997) A phase III comparison of two toremifene doses to tamoxifen in postmenopausal women with advanced breast cancer. Eastern European Study Group. Breast Cancer Res Treat 45:251–262

Geyer CE, Forster J, Lindquist S, et al. (2006) Lapatinib plus capecitabine for HER 2 positive advanced breast cancer. NEJM 355:2733–2743

Gradishar WJ, Tjulandin S, Davidson N, et al. (2005) Phase III trial of nanoparticle albumin-bound paclitaxel compared with polyethylated castor oil-based paclitaxel in women with breast cancer. J Clin Oncol 23:7794–7803

Hayes DF, Zyl Van JA, Hacking A, et al. (1995) Randomized comparison of tamoxifen and two separate doses of toremifene in postmenopausal patients with metastatic breast cancer. J Clin Oncol 13:2556–2566

Klijn JG, Beex LV, Mauriac L, et al. (2000) Combined treatment with buserelin and tamoxifen in premenopausal metastatic breast cancer: a randomized study. J Natl Cancer Inst 92:903–911

Marty M, Cognetti F, Maraninchi D, et al. (2005) Randomized phase II trial of the efficacy and safety of trastuzumab combined with docetaxel in patients with human epidermal growth factor receptor

2-positive metastatic breast cancer administered as first-line treatment: the M77001 study group. J Clin Oncol 23:4265–4274

Miller K, Wang M, Gralow J, et al. (2007) Paclitaxel plus bevacizumab versus paclitaxel alone for metastatic breast cancer. NEJM 357:2666–2676

Mouridsen H, Gershanovich M, Sun Y, et al. (2001) Superior efficacy of letrozole versus tamoxifen as first-line therapy for postmenopausal women with advanced breast cancer: results of a phase III study of the International Letrozole Breast Cancer Group. J Clin Oncol 19:2596–2606

Nabholtz JM, Buzdar A, Pollak M, et al. (2000) Anastrozole is superior to tamoxifen as first-line therapy for advanced breast cancer in post-menopausal women: results of a North American multicenter randomized trial. Arimidex Study Group. J Clin Oncol 18:3758–3767

O'Shaughnessy J, Miles D, Vukelja S, et al. (2002) Superior survival with capecitabine plus docetaxel combination therapy in anthracycline-pretreated patients with advanced breast cancer: phase III trial results. J Clin Oncol 20:2812–2823

Paridaens R, Therasse P, Dirix L, Dirix L (2004) First line hormonal treatment (HT) for metastatic breast cancer (MBC) with exemestane (E) or tamoxifen (T) in postmenopausal patients (pts) -A randomized phase III trial of the EORTC Breast Group. Journal of Clinical Oncology, 2004 ASCO Annual Meeting Proceedings 22(14S):A515

Pyrhonen S, Valavaara R, Modig H, et al. (1997) Comparison of tore-mifene and tamoxifen in post-menopausal patients with advanced breast cancer: a randomized double-blind, the "nordic" phase III study. Br J Cancer 76:270–277

Robert N, Leyland-Jones B, Asmar L, et al. (2006) Randomized phase III study of trastuzumab, paclitaxel, and carboplatin compared with trastuzumab and paclitaxel in women with HER-2-overexpressing metastatic breast cancer. J Clin Oncol 24:2786–2792

Slamon DJ, Leyland-Jones B, Shak S, et al. (2001) Use of chemotherapy plus a monoclonal antibody against HER2 for metastatic breast cancer that overexpresses HER2. N Engl J Med 344:783–792

Sledge GW, Neuberg D, Bernardo P, et al. (2003) Phase III trial of doxo-rubicin, paclitaxel, and the combination of doxorubicin and pacli-taxel as front-line chemotherapy for metastatic breast cancer: An intergroup trial (E1193). J Clin Oncol 21:588–592

Vogel CL, Cobleigh MA, Tripathy D, et al. (2002) Efficacy and safety of trastuzumab as a single agent in first-line treatment of HER2-overexpressing metastatic breast cancer. J Clin Oncol 20:719–726

Wilkins EW, Jr., Head JM, Burke JF (1978) Pulmonary resection for metastatic neoplasms in the lung. Experience at the Massachusetts General Hospital. Am J Surg 135:480–483

8
Reconstruction of the Breast

Laurence Z. Rosenberg, Patricio Andrades, and Luis O. Vasconez

Pearls and Pitfalls

- Not all patients are candidates for breast reconstruction.
- There are many options for breast reconstruction; the skilled plastic surgeon does not use a single technique.
- The skin-sparing mastectomy allows for the optimal breast reconstruction.
- Avoid immediate breast reconstruction in patients who are likely to receive radiation.
- Autologous breast reconstruction creates the most natural result, but requires the most extensive operation.
- Avoid implants in obese patients.
- The reconstructed breast is never a perfect replacement for the original breast.

Introduction

Breast reconstruction has advanced significantly over the past 30 years. Current methods of breast reconstruction allow for a natural and aesthetically pleasing reconstruction in most patients. Evidence has demonstrated that breast reconstruction does not interfere with oncologic practice or breast cancer surveillance.

K.I. Bland et al. (eds.), *Surgery in Breast Cancer and Melanoma*, DOI 10.1007/978-1-84996-435-7_8,
© Springer-Verlag London Limited 2011

There are many procedures available for breast reconstruction, and as one examines the list below, the following characteristics should be noted:

1. The technical demand of each procedure increases.
2. The aesthetic result increases.
3. The length of the operation and the recovery time for the patient increases.

Most plastic surgeons cannot offer all forms of breast reconstruction. It is the responsibility of the plastic surgeon to make an appropriate reconstructive recommendation and referral, if necessary.

Presentation

The majority of patients who can tolerate a mastectomy, can tolerate some form of breast reconstruction; the plastic surgeon must match the appropriate operation to the correct patient.

Patients usually present to the plastic surgeon as a referral from the general surgeon who will perform the mastectomy. Reconstruction is the final component of comprehensive management of breast cancer. Reconstruction of the breast should never compromise the cancer treatment.

The site of breast cancer recurrence varies by stage. Stage I breast cancer is most likely to recur locally. Stage II breast cancer is most likely to recur at a distant site (bone). Multiple studies have shown that recurrence is best detected by clinical examination. No study has demonstrated that breast reconstruction affects detection of breast cancer recurrence.

The administration of adjuvant chemotherapy is generally not affected by reconstruction, although postoperative chemotherapy may be delayed if wound complications occur. A prospective study from the University of Alabama at Birmingham comparing 125 patients who underwent immediate breast reconstruction versus 125 who underwent mastectomy alone had the following outcomes: there was no difference in time to initiation of chemotherapy and no difference in complication rate (18%).

Reconstruction should be delayed if postoperative radio-therapy will be recommended. The radiation causes skin changes and results in a less aesthetic result.

Pre-Operative Evaluation

The preoperative consultation allows the patient to meet the plastic surgeon, review the different reconstructive options, and look at photographs of the operative outcomes. The surgeon must listen to the patient and acknowledge her desires. It is imperative that the physician explain to the patient that the reconstructed breast is not a perfect replacement. Also, breast reconstruction requires multiple stages, although the first operation is the longest and requires the longest convalescence.

The preoperative visit also allows the surgeon to decide whether immediate or delayed breast reconstruction should be performed. The final results after immediate reconstruction are aesthetically better, but there are reasons to delay reconstruction, i.e. radiotherapy, advanced breast cancer, and patient preference.

After the decisions are made to perform breast reconstruction and whether an immediate or a delayed operation will be performed, the next decision is which type of reconstruction to perform.

Important factors include the patient's health, smoking history, breast size, obesity, and the patient's desires. As listed in Table 8.1, there are many reconstructive options. The simplest techniques, both for the surgeon to perform and for the patient to tolerate, only use alloplastic material. Currently, there are two types of breast implants: saline-filled silicone shell implants and silicone-cohesive gel implants (Fig. 8.1).

The advantages of reconstruction with an alloplastic implant are:

1. Less operative time.
2. Shorter hospital stay.
3. Quicker recovery.
4. No additional scars elsewhere on the body.

TABLE 8.1. Surgical options for breast reconstruction.

Prosthetic only reconstruction

1. Saline or silicone implant

Autologous and prosthetic reconstruction

2. Thoraco-epigastric flap with implant

3. Latissimus myocutaneous flap with implant

Autologous reconstruction

4. Transverse rectus abdominus myocutaneous flap (TRAM)

5. Extended latissimus myocutaneous flap

6. Free TRAM

7. Deep inferior epigastric artery perforator flap (DIEP)

8. Superficial inferior epigastric artery perforator flap (SIEP)

9. Superior gluteal artery perforator flap (SGAP)

10. Inferior gluteal artery perforator flap (IGAP)

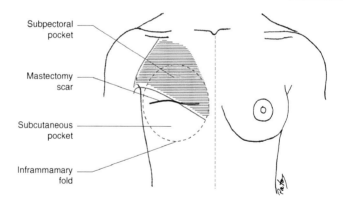

FIGURE 8.1. Implant and expanders reconstruction: for both types of reconstruction, it is recommended to place the device in a submuscular pocket. Unfortunately, the pectoralis major muscle does not cover the lower-third of the implant, even when the serratus anterior muscle is used.

The disadvantages are a less natural feel and a less ideal cosmetic result. Excessive firmness of the breast mound with

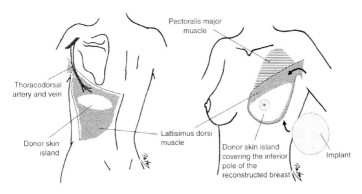

FIGURE 8.2. The latissimus dorsi flap may be used alone to reconstruct a small breast and often requires an implant to rebuild larger
breasts. The skin island may be designed transverse, oblique, or more
vertical in the dorsum. When an implant is used, it should be covered
completely by muscles; sometimes the pectoralis major is necessary.
In delayed reconstruction, the skin island is placed in the inferior
pole of the reconstructed breast, and when it is immediate, the skin
requirements are decreased and limited to the nipple-areola complex area.

possible capsular contraction is also a potential disadvantage.
Capsular contraction is the presence of dense scar tissue
around the implant that may cause firmness, distortion of the
breast, and possibly significant pain.

An intermediate form of breast reconstruction utilizes
both an implant to create volume and a muscle to cover the
implant, so it is not palpable through the skin. The most common
muscle utilized is the latissimus dorsi (Fig. 8.2). This operation is less extensive than autologous-only breast reconstruction. Also, there are minimal scars outside the breast mound,
a more natural result than implant-only reconstruction and,
minimal morbidity for the donor site.

There are many methods for autologous tissue breast
reconstruction. The methods are generally divided in two
groups (Fig. 8.3):

1. Pedicled flap reconstruction.
2. Free flap reconstruction (requires microvascular surgery).

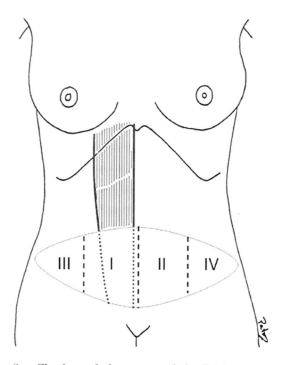

FIGURE 8.3. Classic perfusion zones of the TRAM flap: Zone I (located over the muscle that is going to be used to elevate the flan), Zone II (located over the contralateral muscle; Zone III (located lateral to zone I), and Zone IV (located lateral to zone II). Zone I is the best and zone IV is the worst vascularized, so the areas that must be used for a safe and reliable reconstruction are the central portions of the flap.

Autologous tissue reconstruction results in the most aesthetic and natural-feeling breast reconstruction. The operations take more time to perform, are more technically demanding, and require a longer postoperative convalescence for the patient.

The most common form of autologous tissue reconstruction is the Transverse Rectus Abdominis Myocutaneous flap. This procedure involves transposing the abdominal skin and fat to the chest wall to recreate the breast mound. The blood supply to the tissue may be provided in several ways.

Perforating blood vessels arise from the epigastric system, pass though the rectus abdominis muscle, and supply the skin and soft tissue of the abdomen. In the pedicled TRAM flap, the insertion of the rectus abdominis muscle is divided and the muscle is used as a conduit to carry blood to the flap.

In an effort to preserve the rectus muscle, the flap can be elevated on the inferior epigastric vessels, the dominant blood supply, and transferred to the chest wall. This technique may take a portion of the rectus muscle, a free TRAM, or none at all (Deep Inferior Epigastric Perforator Flap). The TRAM flap takes 3–8 h, depending on the technique.

Secondary Procedures

After the breast mound is reconstructed, nipple reconstruction, areola tattooing (Fig. 8.4), and small revisions are required. The procedures are usually done under local anesthesia or IV sedation.

Complications

Postoperative complications specific to the reconstructive operation are flap loss, donor site breakdown, and poor aesthetic results. As with all surgery, skin necrosis, wound dehiscence, and hematoma are always possible.

Conclusion

Breast reconstruction is an integral part of breast cancer management, and most patients are candidates. It is the responsibility of the plastic surgeon to discuss the reconstructive options with the patient and determine the optimal surgical procedure.

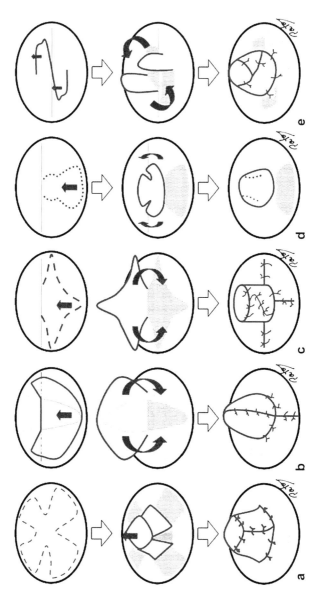

FIGURE 8.4. Nipple reconstruction techniques. **a.** Malta Cruz technique; **b.** skate flap; **c.** star flap; **d.** bell flap; **e.** double-opposing flag flap.

Selected Readings

Bostwick J III (1985) Breast reconstruction following mastectomy. Contemp Surg 27:15

Hietanen P (1986) Relapse pattern and follow-up of breast cancer. Ann Clin Res 18:134

Lee Y (1984) Breast carcinoma: pattern of recurrence and metastasis after mastectomy. Am J Clin Oncol 7:443

Pivot X, et al. (2000) A retrospective study of first indicators of breast cancer recurrence. Oncology 58:185

Roselli Del Turco M, et al. (1994) Intensive diagnostic follow-up after treatment of primary breast cancer: a randomized trial. National Research Council Project on Breast Cancer follow-up. JAMA 271:1593

Slavin SA, Love SM, Goldwyn RM (1994) Recurrent breast cancer following immediate reconstruction with myocutaneous flaps. Plast Reconstr Surg 93:1191

Wilkins EG, et al. (2001) Prospective analysis of psychosocial outcomes in breast reconstruction: one-year postoperative results from the Michigan Breast Reconstruction Outcome Study. Clin Plast Surg 28:435

Part II
Skin Soft Tissues

9
Evaluation of Malignant and Premalignant Skin Lesions

Kelly M. McMasters

Pearls and Pitfalls

- Skin examination should be a routine part of the physical examination.
- Biopsy any concerning skin lesion that the patient has brought to your attention, unless it is unequivocally benign.
- It is easier to biopsy a suspicious skin lesion than to follow it clinically.
- Use the ABCDE acronym for melanoma to evaluate suspicious pigmented lesions.
- Teach prevention at every opportunity: avoid excessive sun exposure, wear protective clothing, avoid tanning beds.
- Patients with significant solar damage to the skin, or with premalignant or malignant skin lesions should be followed by a dermatologist.

Introduction

Examination of the skin should be a regular component of the physical examination. Although a detailed dermatologic examination, with photography and measurement of all skin lesions, may be beyond the scope of most primary care physicians, a complete skin survey to detect suspicious lesions

K.I. Bland et al. (eds.), *Surgery in Breast Cancer and Melanoma*, DOI 10.1007/978-1-84996-435-7_9,
© Springer-Verlag London Limited 2011

takes about 1 min and can be life-saving. It requires no special equipment, and can be performed in any physician's office. It requires the simplest of preparation: that the patient be undressed. All physicians should be aware of the basics of evaluation of skin lesions to detect early premalignant and malignant lesions.

In this chapter, the characteristics of a variety of common skin lesions will be reviewed. Please be aware, however, that many skin cancers can present in an atypical fashion. Some general rules apply to evaluation of all skin lesions. First, no skin lesion is definitively diagnosed without a biopsy. All physicians should know the basics of performing a biopsy of a suspicious lesion. Any non-healing skin lesion, regardless of appearance, should be biopsied. Any lesion that has grown or changed over time should be biopsied. Whenever a patient brings a lesion to the attention of the physician because it itches, bleeds, has changed in size or color, or because they are concerned about it, the simplest and easiest approach is to perform a biopsy. While many benign lesions such as seborrheic keratoses can be safely observed, it is astounding how often patients present to a physician with a complaint of a skin lesion that concerns them, are told to "keep an eye on it," and later are diagnosed with skin cancer. Like a complete skin survey, a biopsy takes about 1 min. Many times I have had a similar experience: I evaluated a patient's skin lesion, told them I thought it looked benign and should be observed, walked out of the patient's room, then had a nagging feeling that I should perform a biopsy. I then performed a biopsy and diagnosed a skin cancer. I have learned that it is easier to perform a biopsy than to worry about it.

Skin Biopsy

A skin biopsy involves removal of a small portion of abnormal skin to be evaluated by a pathologist. There are three main types of skin biopsies, excisional (or incisional), punch, and shave biopsy. All are performed after injection of local anesthetic. An excisional biopsy is performed with an elliptical or fusiform incision to excise the lesion completely, then closing the defect with sutures. An incisional biopsy is the same except that only a portion of the lesion is excised; this is most commonly performed when the lesion is larger than about 1.5 cm or if complete excision would be difficult to achieve with good cosmetic outcome, yet tissue diagnosis is required. A punch biopsy uses a disposable cookie cutter-like tool to remove a cylindrical portion of the lesion. This is usually closed with a suture or two. Punch biopsy instruments (Fig. 9.1) come in a variety of sizes ranging from 2 to 8 mm in diameter. In general, it is best to use a larger punch (6 mm is ideal) to provide the pathologist with adequate tissue for diagnosis. Multiple punch biopsies of larger skin lesions can be performed. In general, the punch should be through the thickest portion of the skin lesion; there is no advantage to biopsy at the junction of the lesion with normal skin. Excisional, incisional, and punch biopsies should remove a portion of skin with underlying subcutaneous tissue to achieve a full-thickness skin biopsy. A shave biopsy is performed using a scalpel or razor blade-like instrument to

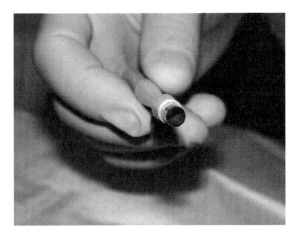

FIGURE 9.1. Punch biopsy instrument.

shave a partial thickness biopsy of the skin beneath the lesion. This can be accomplished by passing a needle (21–25 gauge) beneath the lesion and shaving beneath the lesion. A deep shave or saucerization biopsy is a technique to remove a deeper, often full-thickness, portion of the skin. Shave biopsy is attractive because it is very rapid and does not require suturing of the skin – hemostasis is achieved by direct pressure, or by chemical means (aluminum chloride, silver nitrate), or by the use of cautery. The patient then applies antibiotic ointment to the site twice per day, which will heal in about 1–2 weeks.

Shave biopsy is usually discouraged for pigmented lesions because it is possible to shave directly through a melanoma. Cauterization of the base can then distort the final pathology reading, resulting in underestimation of the true thickness of a melanoma. However, in the hands of experienced dermatologists and other clinicians, a deep shave or saucerization biopsy can be a very useful technique. Of course, a shave biopsy is better than no biopsy at all if it means the difference between early and late diagnosis of a skin cancer.

Seborrheic Keratosis

Seborrheic keratoses are benign and very common pigmented papular skin lesions that can have the appearance of wart-like growths on the surface of the skin (Fig. 9.2). They are often waxy or rough and wart-like, with a "pasted on" appearance, such that they look as if they could be scraped off with a fingernail. They often appear after age 40, can appear all over the body, and have been described as the "barnacles of life" because they develop so commonly as patients age. Seborrheic keratoses can appear in large numbers. They can have a variety of colors, but often are tan, gray, or brown. They are usually painless and benign, but may become irritated and itch. Most seborrheic keratoses are easily diagnosed by their appearance and do not require biopsy. However, even experienced dermatologists are occasionally fooled by a melanoma that presents with the appearance of a

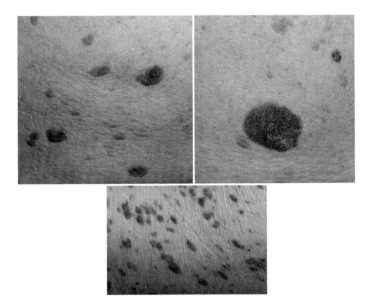

FIGURE 9.2. Seborrheic keratoses (Courtesy of Dr. Timothy Brown, Louisville, KY).

seborrheic keratosis. Other skin cancers may be diagnosed either adjacent to or within a seborrheic keratosis as well. If treatment is needed, seborrheic keratoses may be surgically removed or treated with cryotherapy.

Actinic Keratosis

Actinic keratoses are precancerous skin lesions usually caused by sun exposure. They occur most commonly as macular rough lesions in patients with fair skin, especially in the elderly and in younger individuals with light complexions. They occur in sun-exposed skin areas. Actinic keratoses begin as flat, scaly areas that are often pink, erythematous, or flesh-colored (Fig. 9.3). They later develop a hard, gritty, rough or wart-like surface. If left untreated, approximately 1% of actinic keratoses develop into squamous cell carcinoma.

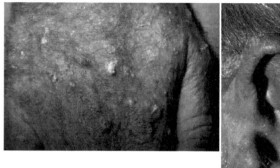
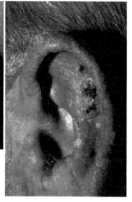

FIGURE 9.3. Actinic keratoses (Courtesy of Dr. Timothy Brown).

Biopsy is indicated if squamous cell carcinoma is suspected; however, usually actinic keratoses can be treated with non-surgical means such as cryotherapy, electrical cautery, or with topical agents such as 5-fluorouracil or imiquimod.

Basal Cell Carcinoma

Basal cell carcinoma is the most common form of skin cancer. It accounts for about 75% of all skin cancers, with an annual incidence of approximately 400,000–500,000 patients in the USA. More than 90% of basal cell carcinomas occur on areas of the skin that are regularly exposed to sunlight or other ultraviolet radiation. Basal cell carcinomas are more common in those who have fair skin, blue or green eyes, and blonde or red hair. The onset most commonly occurs after age 40. These are usually papular but can be macular lesions with a pearly or waxy appearance. They can be white, pink, or flesh-colored, sometimes with visible blood vessels in the lesion or the adjacent skin (Fig. 9.4). A new skin lesion that ulcerates, bleeds easily, or a non-healing sore may indicate development of basal cell skin carcinoma. They are commonly found in

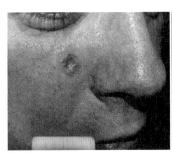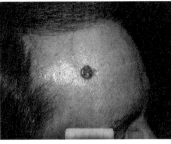

FIGURE 9.4. Basal cell carcinoma (Courtesy of Dr. Timothy Brown).

sun-exposed areas such as the face, scalp, ear, neck, chest, back, arms, and hands. Most basal cell carcinomas are easily cured, and do not metastasize. However, if neglected, these cancers can cause significant morbidity, especially with extensive invasion around the eyes, nose, and ears. Biopsy is required to make a definitive diagnosis. The treatment varies depending on the size, depth, and location of the cancer. Curettage, cryosurgery, cauterization, excision, or Mohs surgery are the preferred methods of treatment.

Squamous Cell Carcinoma

Squamous cell carcinoma is the other common form of skin cancer that usually is slow growing and easily treated. However, squamous cell carcinoma has the potential to metastasize to lymph nodes and other organs, especially when the tumors are large and poorly differentiated. It can be particularly aggressive in immunosuppressed individuals. Squamous cell carcinoma affects approximately 150,000 patients per year in the USA. Like basal cell carcinoma, squamous cell carcinoma usually develops in chronically sun-exposed areas of the body, especially on the face, ears, neck, hands and arms and is more common in people with fair skin. It may arise from areas of actinic keratosis, and usually appears after the age of 50. It usually presents as a macular or papular red, crusted or

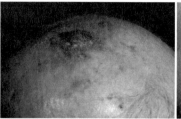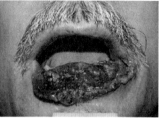

FIGURE 9.5. Squamous cell carcinoma (Courtesy of Dr. Timothy Brown).

scaly lesion and as it progresses often forms a non-healing ulcer (Fig. 9.5). Biopsy is indicated for diagnosis. Treatment options depend on the size, location, and depth of the tumor, and include surgical excision with negative margins and Mohs surgery. Squamous cell carcinoma is curable in over 95% of cases with surgical excision, but patients must be followed closely as they are prone to develop other skin cancers.

Melanoma

Melanoma is the most serious form of skin cancer, as it is more likely than other common skin cancers to metastasize to lymph nodes and other organs. Approximately 60,000 new melanomas are diagnosed each year in the USA, and the incidence has risen faster than any other malignancy. The estimated lifetime incidence of melanoma is now 1 in 53 for men and 1 in 78 for women in the USA. Risk factors include fair skin, blonde or red hair, blue or green eyes, 3 or more years spent at an outdoor summer job as a teenager, obvious freckling on the upper back and chest, and a history of severe sunburns or excessive sun exposure, particularly among patients with three or more episodes of blistering sunburns before age 20. Mounting evidence also implicates tanning bed use in the development of not only basal cell and squamous cell carcinoma, but melanoma as well.

Melanoma can develop de novo, or within an existing nevus. Early detection provides the best chance for cure. The ABCDEs of melanoma are used for diagnosis:

Asymmetric: irregularly shaped lesion

Borders: irregular or scalloped borders

Color: variegated color, often with various shades of black, brown, tan, red, blue, gray

Diameter: usually greater than 6 mm, although the incidence of melanomas detected less than 6 mm in diameter has increased

Evolution: any skin lesion that changes over time, itches, bleeds, or ulcerates

While the ABCDEs provide a useful framework for diagnosis, atypical presentation of melanoma is common. Many patients are now diagnosed with amelanotic lesions that may have the appearance of a pink or flesh-colored lesion that grows over time. Biopsy is indicated for any non-healing lesion, or any that change in size, color, shape, as well as those that itch, bleed, or ulcerate. A patient's history of a rapidly growing lesion is sufficient to warrant a biopsy (Fig. 9.6).

There are four main histological subtypes of melanoma: superficial spreading melanoma, nodular, lentigo maligna melanoma, and acral. Superficial spreading melanoma is the most common type of melanoma. It is usually flat and irregular in shape and color, with varying shades of black and brown. Nodular melanoma presents as a papular lesion that may or may not be darkly pigmented. Lentigo maligna melanoma most commonly is found in elderly patients, often on the face, but also on the neck and arms. It often presents as a flat, irregular pigmented lesion, and negative margins may be difficult to achieve initially because the extent of the microscopically tumor-involved skin may be greater than the area of visible abnormal pigmentation. Acral lentiginous melanoma is found on the palms of the hands, soles of the feet, and under the nails (subungual melanoma). These lesions often present at an advanced stage. Subungual melanomas are often mistaken for a subungual hematoma, with a resulting

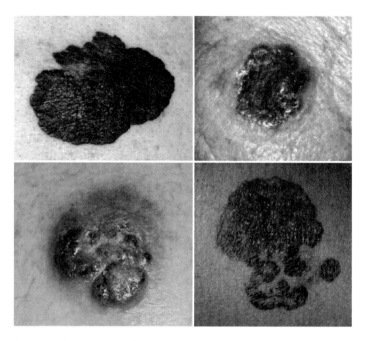

FIGURE 9.6. Melanoma (Courtesy of Dr. Timothy Brown).

delay in diagnosis. Any dark pigmentation that does not grow out as the nail grows should be considered suspicious for subungual melanoma. Subungual lesions can be biopsied by performing a digital block, removing the nail, and performing a punch or incisional biopsy. Alternatively, a punch biopsy can be performed directly through the nail.

Dysplastic Nevi

Dysplastic nevi are pigmented lesions that can potentially progress to melanoma. The ABCDEs of melanoma often will detect dysplastic nevi as well. Dysplastic nevi often are irregular, asymmetric, with irregular borders; variable colors including black, brown, tan, red, and pink; often are at least 5 mm in size; and may change over time. Approximately 4% of the population has dysplastic nevi. Dysplastic nevus-melanoma syndrome refers to the presence of multiple dysplastic nevi and melanoma in two or more first-degree relatives. Such patients with dysplastic nevi are at an increased risk of developing melanoma. Dysplastic nevi may occur anywhere on the body but most frequently are found on the back and in sun-exposed areas.

Prevention

Skin cancer prevention relies on avoidance and protection from the damaging effects of ultraviolet (UV) radiation. Unfortunately, a large amount of UV radiation damage is intentional among those who sunbathe and use tanning beds. Recommendations include wearing protective clothing, including hats, long sleeves, and sunglasses, avoidance of sunbathing and tanning beds, frequent application of sunblock that contains agents that provide both UVA and UVB protection with a sun protection factor (SPF) of 15 or higher, and refraining from sun exposure during the peak hours of 10:00 AM and 2:00 PM. Those with fair skin must be particularly vigilant because a severe sunburn can occur within a very short time of intense sun exposure. The growing use of tanning beds among children and teenagers is a worrisome trend, as many patients with skin cancer are now diagnosed at a young age.

Selected Readings

Berman B, Bienstock L, Kuritzky L, et al. (2006) Actinic keratoses: sequelae and treatments. Recommendations from a consensus panel. J Fam Pract 55(Suppl):1–8

Cummins DL, Cummins JM, Pantle H, et al. (2006) Cutaneous malignant melanoma. Mayo Clin Proc 81:500–507

Jemal A, Murray T, Ward E, et al. (2005) Cancer statistics, 2005. CA Cancer J Clin 55:10–30

Lim C (2006) Seborrhoeic keratoses with associated lesions: a retrospective analysis of 85 lesions. Australasian J Dermatology 47:109–113

Nguyen TH, Ho DQ (2002) Nonmelanoma skin cancer. Curr Treat Options Oncol 3:193–203

Zuber TJ (2002) Punch biopsy of the skin. Am Fam Physician 65:1155–1158

10
Staging and Treatment Options for Cutaneous Melanoma

Julie R. Lange, Ajay Jain, Glen C. Balch, and Charles M. Balch

Pearls and Pitfalls

- Biopsy of lesions suspicious for melanoma must be full-thickness.
- The measured tumor thickness, the presence or absence of ulceration on histologic review, and the number of metastatic lymph nodes are the most important prognostic features of melanoma.
- In the absence of symptoms or signs of metastatic disease, the preoperative evaluation of a patient newly diagnosed with clinical stage I or II melanoma should be limited to physical exam, chest x-ray and serum liver function tests including lactate dehydrogenase.
- Indications for sentinel node biopsy include primary invasive melanoma ≥1 mm in thickness with no evidence of regional or distant metastases, or primary melanoma < 1 mm with the risk features such as ulceration or Clark's level IV.
- Sentinel node biopsy should be done before the wide local excision.
- The number of metastatic lymph nodes and the tumor burden are the dominant predictors of survival in patients with Stage III melanoma.
- A thin shave biopsy of lesions suspicious for melanoma should be avoided as this may compromise the histologic interpretation and proper measurement of the thickness.

K.I. Bland et al. (eds.), *Surgery in Breast Cancer and Melanoma*, DOI 10.1007/978-1-84996-435-7_10,
© Springer-Verlag London Limited 2011

- The sentinel node(s) should be placed in formalin for permanent fixation. It is preferable to save the lymph node intact for permanent processing only, so that multiple sections can be taken with immunohistochemical stains (HMB-45, S-100, Melan-A) to look for microscopic evidence of disease.
- It is unnecessary to obtain CT scans or PET scans except for patients with Stage IV melanoma and in selected patients with Stage IIIB/C melanoma.

Introduction

The incidence of cutaneous melanoma has increased over the past four decades. In 2008, there will be an estimated 62,480 new cases of cutaneous melanoma and 8,420 melanoma-related deaths in the United States. At the time of diagnosis 80–85% of patients have localized disease only, 10–13% have regional disease and 2–5% have distant metastasis. Surgery remains the mainstay of treatment for melanoma in patients with local or regional disease. In localized melanoma, surgery alone is often curative. For patients with regional disease other treatment modalities may be considered in conjunction with surgical resection. The goals of surgery in melanoma patients are locoregional control, nodal staging and in most cases potential for cure.

Fortunately, most melanoma patients are diagnosed at an early stage today and are usually curable with surgery alone. When considering the proper management of cutaneous melanoma, the importance of staging cannot be over-emphasized. The complexity of the staging system for cutaneous melanoma is based on data that correlates features of the primary tumor and the presence of locoregional or distant metastases with long term prognosis. Wide local excision provides local control of the primary tumor site, but does not address occult metastatic disease that may be present. Lymphatic mapping and sentinel node biopsy may be considered for many patients with newly diagnosed melanoma as a staging procedure. This chapter reviews the diagnosis and evaluation of patients with melanoma, the current staging system, and the rationale for selecting treatment options.

Clinical Presentation and Biopsy

Cutaneous melanoma can arise anywhere on the body. The most common site in women is the lower extremity and the most common site in men is the back. Clinical features typical of melanoma include variegated color, irregular borders or a history of a change in such as a skin lesion. A simple mnemonic to remember concerning features of a pigmented lesion is "ABCDE." The concerning features are **A**symmetry, **B**order irregularity, **C**olor change/variegation, **D**iameter change, and **E**volution (change over time) of the lesion. Some melanomas do not have typical features; some are non-pigmented and may resemble other dermatologic findings such as basal cell carcinoma, squamous cell carcinoma, seborrheic keratosis or dermatofibroma. Individuals at notably increased risk of melanoma are those with a prior history of melanoma, a family history of melanoma, a high number(>20) of benign moles, atypical moles or congenital nevi.

Proper biopsy of a suspicious lesion is critical to proper staging. Suspicious lesions should have a full-thickness biopsy in order to accurately interpret the maximum tumor thickness, the presence or absence of ulceration and the level of invasion. Excisional biopsy with a narrow margin of normal-appearing skin for small lesions is preferred; this can be performed on most small lesions. The biopsy scar should be oriented to be compatible with a subsequent wide local excision if the lesion proves to be melanoma. Incisional biopsy (usually a punch biopsy) is appropriate for lesions which are large (e.g., >1.5 cm) or which are at a vital anatomic site where one would want to know the diagnosis before removing the entire lesion (e.g., face or hands). Incisional biopsy should be performed at the most raised area, but since it removes only part of a tumor, a repeat biopsy maybe necessary if the histologic diagnosis does not agree with the clinical impression. Final determination of the tumor thickness cannot be made until the entire lesion has been excised, sectioned, and examined by the dermatopathologist. Although punch biopsy is often appropriate, a thin shave biopsy of lesions suspicious for melanoma should be avoided as this can compromise the histologic interpretation and proper measurement of thickness.

The primary lesion should be reviewed by an experienced dermatopathologist to confirm the diagnosis. Microstaging with an ocular micrometer measures the maximum tumor thickness. The presence or absence of ulceration should be specifically commented upon. Other features of the primary tumor worth noting include level of invasion, mitotic rate, degree of regression (if any), and presence of tumor-infiltrating lymphocytes. The pathologic report of the melanoma is the primary document from which clinical decisions are made.

Melanoma: AJCC Staging

Staging of melanoma combines those clinical and pathologic features of melanoma that best predict survival outcome of a patient. Patients with a localized invasive melanoma are categorized as Stage I or II (depending on the thickness). The presence of regional nodal metastases upstages the patient to Stage III regardless of the thickness of the primary tumor. The presence of distant metastases indicates Stage IV disease. In 2003, the Melanoma Task Force of the American Joint Committee on Cancer (AJCC) revised the melanoma staging system. Although this staging system is complex, it is a very powerful tool that partitions melanoma patients into homogeneous risk groups based on the probability of harboring occult metastatic disease. This, in turn, allows the surgeon to determine how to proceed with diagnostic evaluation, surgical therapy and nodal staging, and recommendations for adjuvant systemic treatments. These prognostic and staging criteria are also essential in the design, analysis and comparison of melanoma clinical trials.

The 2003 staging system has basic features of a standard TNM staging system:

- A primary tumor in the absence of nodal or regional metastases indicates Stage I or II disease (depending upon tumor thickness)
- The presence of regional metastases indicates Stage III disease
- Distant metastasis indicates Stage IV disease

Within each stage, there are separate substages that are determined by pathologic features of the primary melanoma or the volume of nodal or regional disease. These features are significant determinants of prognosis.

The 2003 AJCC staging system is summarized in Tables 10.1 and 10.2 Tumor thickness is made the most important aspect of T staging. Level of invasion (Clark's level) only has prognostic significance in thin(T1) melanomas. The thickness of a melanoma (Breslow thickness, as measured with an ocular micrometer) may be related to the rate of growth and/or the duration of the lesions. The risk of nodal and distant metastases increases linearly with the tumor thickness. Thin lesions (less than 1 mm thick) generally have a low risk of nodal spread, and most thin melanomas can be managed with wide local excision alone.

Tumor ulceration (microscopic interruption of the surface epithelium by tumor) is recognized as a poor prognostic factor. When the primary melanoma is ulcerated the risk of nodal metastases is greater for all tumor thickness groups. Within a tumor stage, the presence of ulceration raises the substage from a to b (Example: Anon-ulcerated 0.5 mm melanoma is stage Ia, but an ulcerated melanoma of the same thickness is Stage Ib). In some instances, ulceration can raise the staging by a whole stage level. For example, a 1.5 mm, non-ulcerated melanoma without nodal metastases (T2, N0) is classified as Stage Ib. The presence of ulceration in the same lesion raises the stage to IIa. In a prognostic factor analysis from The University of Texas MD Anderson Cancer Center and the Moffitt Cancer Center, thickness and ulceration were the two most powerful predictors of microscopic nodal metastasis detected by sentinel lymphadenectomy.

TABLE 10.1. Melanoma TNM classification.

T classification	Thickness	Ulceration status
TI	1 mm	a: w/o ulceration and level II/III b: with ulceration or level IV/V
T2	1.01–2 mm	a: w/o ulceration b: with ulceration
T3	2.01–4 mm	a: w/o ulceration b: with ulceration
T4	>4 mm	a: w/o ulceration b: with ulceration
N classification	**# of Metastatic nodes**	**Nodal metastatic mass**
N1	1 node	a: micrometastasis[a] b: macrometastasis[b]
N2	2–3 nodes	a: micrometastasis[a] b: macrometastasis[b] c: in transit met(s)/ satellite(s) without metastatic nodes
N3	4 or more metastatic nodes or matted nodes, or in transit met(s)/satellite(s) and metastatic node(s)	
M classification	**Site**	**Serum LDH**
M1	Distant skin, SQ or nodal mets	Normal
M2	Lung metastases	Normal
	All other visceral metastases	Normal
M3	Or any distant metastasis	Elevated

[a]Micrometastases are diagnosed after elective or sentinel lymphadenectomy.
[b]Macrometastases are defined as clinically detectable nodal metastases confirmed by therapeutic lymphadenectomy or when nodal metastasis exhibits gross extracapsular extension.

TABLE 10.2. Stage groupings for cutaneous melanoma.

Clinical staging[a]				Pathologic staging[b]			
0	Tis	N0	M0	**0**	Tis	N0	M0
IA	T1a	N0	M0	**IA**	T1a	N0	M0
IB	T1b	N0	M0	**IB**	T1b	N0	M0
	T2a	N0	M0		T2a	N0	M0
IIA	T2b	N0	M0	**IIA**	T2b	N0	M0
	T3a	N0	M0		T3a	N0	M0
IIB	T3b	N0	M0	**IIB**	T3b	N0	M0
	T4a	N0	M0		T4a	N0	M0
IIC	T4b	N0	M0	**IIC**	T4b	N0	M0
IIIA	Any T	N1	M0	**IIIA**	T1–4a	N1a	M0
					T1–4a	N2a	M0
IIIB	Any T	N (multiple)	M0	**IIIB**	T1–4b	N1a	M0
					T1–4b	N2a	M0
					T1–4a	N1b	M0
					T1–4a	N2b	M0
					T1–4a/b	N2c	M0
IIIC	Any T	N satellite(s)	M0	**IIIC**	T1–4b	N1b	M0
					T1–4b	N2b	M0
	Any T	N in-transit(s)	M0		Any T	N3	M0
IV	Any T	any N	Any M	**IV**	Any T	Any N	Any M

[a]Clinical staging includes microstaging of the primary melanoma and clinical/radiologic evaluation for metastases. By convention, it should be used after complete excision of the primary melanoma with clinical assessment for regional and distant metastases.

[b]Pathologic staging includes microstaging of the primary melanoma and pathologic information about the regional lymph nodes after partial or complete lymphadenectomy. Pathologic Stage 0 or Stage 1A patients are the exception; they do not need pathologic evaluation of their lymph nodes.

Patients with nodal metastases have Stage III disease. The number of involved lymph nodes is the strongest predictor of outcome, regardless of whether the patient has macroscopic or microscopic nodal metastases. In all studies that have examined prognosis based upon the number of metastatic nodes, patients with one metastatic node did better than did patients with two or more metastatic nodes. The diameter of nodal metastases does not factor into the current staging system; however the distinction between microscopic (not clinically apparent, such as those found at sentinel node biopsy) and macroscopic (clinically apparent) does affect stage and prognosis. Any amount of tumor seen under the microscope that cannot be detected clinically is defined as micrometastatic disease. As sentinel node mapping and selective lymphadenectomy have become more common, more patients are being identified with clinically occult (microscopic) nodal disease. Patients with microscopic nodal involvement fare better compared to those who have a clinically evident nodal metastases. Patients with intralymphatic metastases, such as satellite metastases located around the primary melanoma or in transit metastases, are recognized as being in a risk category similar to patients with nodal metastases and are thus recognized in the staging system as either N2 or N3 disease, depending on whether nodal metastases are also present.

Finally, some changes were also made in the staging of patients with advanced melanoma. Previously, all patients with visceral metastases were grouped in the same risk category. It is now believed that patients with lung metastases have a lower risk than patients with other visceral metastases. Additionally, elevation of LDH levels are considered negative prognostic indicator in patients with metastatic disease. The 2003 TNM classification is displayed in Table 10.1. Stage groupings are in Table 10.2.

Prognosis

At the time of diagnosis of primary melanoma a number of clinical features and pathological features other than thickness and ulceration are also known to be associated with prognosis. Recent studies have shown that the mitotic rate of a primary melanoma is an important and independent predictor of outcome. Level of invasion into the dermis (in melanoma <1mm) and histologic growth pattern of the primary lesion have some prognostic significance. Superficial spreading and nodular melanoma are the most common histologic types, together constituting more than 85–90% of all melanomas; these two types have approximately the same prognostic significance when matched for tumor thickness. Lentigo maligna melanoma has a more favorable prognosis, whereas in general, acral lentiginous melanoma and desmoplastic melanoma have a worse prognosis. Some anatomic sites of melanoma are associated with increased risk of recurrence, especially the head and neck. Next in frequency of recurrence are trunk melanomas; less likely to recur are extremity melanomas. Older age is associated with higher risk of recurrence, with patients 60 years of age or older at greater risk than patients younger than sixty.

When considering specific prognostic predictors relating to an individual case, it is helpful to consider the primary tumor, and whether nodal, satellite, distant, metastases are present. Tumor thickness and ulceration remain the most important prognostic features of the primary melanoma. Thicker primary tumor or the presence of histologic ulceration implies a greatly increased risk of local, regional, and distant recurrence following surgical excision. However, the status of the regional lymph nodes is the single most important feature in predicting overall survival. If regional lymph nodes are involved the 5-year survival is substantially lower than if the nodes are negative. Prognosis worsens as the number of tumor bearing nodes increases, and patients with macroscopic tumor burden in regional lymph nodes have a worse prognosis than those with micrometastatic disease. The presence of ulceration of the primary tumor retains prognostic significance in node positive patients. Table 10.3 shows the wide range of prognoses in patients with node-positive melanoma.

Patients with melanoma metastases beyond the regional node basin have Stage IV disease and a poor overall prognosis. Some features of the metastatic findings are associated with differing prognoses within the Stage IV group. Metastases in the skin, subcutaneous tissues, or even distant lymph nodes

TABLE 10.3. Five-year survival rates for melanoma patients with nodal metastases, stratified for nodal tumor burden, number of positive nodes, and ulceration of the primary (From Balch et al., 2001b. Reprinted with permission from the American Society of Clinical Oncology).

Number of positive nodes and tumor burden	Non-ulcerated Primary		Ulcerated Primary	
	% ± SE	No.	% ± SE	No.
Microscopic involvement				
1	69 ± 3.7	252	52 ± 4.1	217
23	63 ± 5.6	130	50 ± 5.7	111
≥ 4	27 ± 9.3	57	37 ± 8.8	46
Macroscopic involvement				
1	59 ± 4.7	122	29 ± 5.0	98
23	46 ± 5.5	93	25 ± 4.4	109
≥ 4	27 ± 4.6	109	13 ± 3.5	104

SE = standard error

are considered to be more favorable than metastases in other locations (such as visceral metastases). In patients with visceral metastases, those with metastases confined only to the lung have a better prognosis than patients with metastases in other organs. Prognosis also worsens as the number of distant metastases increases. Finally, elevation of serum LDH levels is considered a poor prognostic sign in patients with metastatic disease. Figure 10.1 displays 15-year overall survival in patients with Stage I, II, III, IV disease.

Preoperative Evaluation

A careful physical exam with attention toward the skin, regional nodal basins and subcutaneous tissues is the most important element of the evaluation of a patient with newly diagnosed primary cutaneous melanoma. Satellite lesions and in transit lesions should be sought by careful inspection

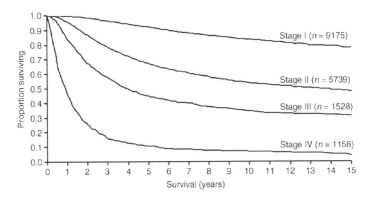

FIGURE 10.1. Fifteen-year survival curves for Stages I, II, III, and IV melanoma. For each curve n = the number of patients in the AJCC melanoma database used to calculate rates. Curve differences are all highly significant (p < 0.0001) (Reprinted from Balch et al., 2001a. Reprinted with permission from the American Society of Clinical Oncology).

of the skin surrounding the primary site and inspection and palpation of subcutaneous tissues between the primary site and the regional nodal basin. The regional nodal basin should be palpated carefully for evidence of nodal metastases. A thorough dermatologic evaluation is important: at least 5% of patients with newly diagnosed melanoma will be found to have another dermatologic malignancy upon careful inspection, either a second melanoma or a basal cell carcinoma or a squamous cell carcinoma.

In the absence of any physical findings or complaints suggestive of regional or distant metastatic disease, the initial evaluation of patients with primary invasive melanoma ≥1mm can be limited to standard chest x-ray and liver function tests including LDH. If these are normal no further preoperative testing is warranted, especially in patients with favorable primary tumors. If preoperative lab work or radiologic studies are abnormal, or if metastatic disease is suspected based on symptoms or clinical findings, then additional diagnostic imaging studies are warranted as dictated by the findings. For patients with questionable palpable adenopathy, ultrasound can define the size and texture of regional lymph nodes and provide radiologic targeting with fine needle aspiration. Suspicious nodal features include loss of the normal oval shape of lymph node to a more rounded contour, disruption or change in morphology of the nodal hilum, cortical thickening of the node, and focal low-level echoes with increased vascularity. Although nodal ultrasound and FNA may occasionally be useful for detecting occult nodal metastases, its sensitivity is limited. If ultrasound-guided FNA is positive, this finding spares the patient a sentinel node biopsy and allows the surgeon to proceed with nodal basin clearance. However, ultrasound can fail to detect abnormalities in a significant percentage of patients with occult nodal disease. A negative preoperative nodal ultrasound does not obviate the staging value of sentinel lymph node biopsy in patients with primary tumor ≥1 mm thick.

If distant metastatic disease is suspected on the basis of concerning symptoms, abnormal chest x-ray or liver enzymes, there are several additional diagnostic tests that may be helpful. Hepatic metastases of melanoma are often hypervascular, and arterial phase computerized tomography (CT) scan imaging may be useful in detecting them. Magnetic resonance imaging (MRI) can be useful for detecting hepatic metastases, and melanoma metastases tend to enhance on T1 weighted imaging. In patients with known positive inguinal nodes, a pelvic CT scan can be used to evaluate the iliac nodes. A standard bone scan can be used when skeletal metastases are suspected. Finally, the use of PET (Positron Emission Tomography) or combined PET-CT may be useful for further evaluating subtle abnormalities noted on standard CT scan. PET imaging might also pick up additional foci of tumor metastases in areas that might otherwise be missed on standard CT. As with other imaging studies, there are limitations in resolution of PET-CT imaging; lesions less than 7 mm in size are expected to be missed on this modality. The role of PET-CT imaging in melanoma is evolving, and at this point is best used for patients with specific diagnostic dilemmas and not for routine screening.

Lymphatic Mapping and Sentinel Node Biopsy

Lymphatic mapping and sentinel node biopsy has emerged over the past decade, and has already significantly altered the surgical approach to primary melanoma in most centers. Initially described by Morton et al., sentinel lymphadenectomy is a highly accurate, minimally invasive method of identifying those primary melanoma patients who may have clinically occult nodal metastases. The technique is based on the now well-supported hypothesis that lymphatic metastases of melanoma follow an orderly progression through afferent lymphatic channels to sentinel lymph nodes before spreading into other regional, non-sentinel lymph nodes. Most experts recommend lymphatic mapping and sentinel lymphadenectomy as a staging procedure for patients with clinical Stage I or II melanoma if their primary tumor is at least 1 mm thick, or, if thinner, when the tumor has high risk features such as ulcerated or is Clark's level IV or V. The lymph node status has important prognostic and clinical implications. Patients found to be node positive are then classified as having Stage III melanoma. Standard therapy is a lymphadenectomy of that nodal basin; these patients can be considered for systemic adjuvant therapy. Knowledge of the nodal status is also important for appropriate stratification of patients who are being considered for entry into a clinical trial. In general, lymphatic mapping and sentinel node biopsy is used for most patients with T1b, T2, T3, or T4 melanomas and a clinically negative regional node basin because the morbidity of the sentinel node procedure is low and the information gained is valuable.

Morton and colleagues reported the results of a randomized prospective study of 1,269 patients with intermediate thickness melanomas (1.2–3.5 mm). They demonstrated that the sentinel node biopsy provides important prognostic information and identifies patients with nodal metastases whose disease control can be improved by lymphadenectomy. This is the first randomized trial to directly assess the staging value of SLN biopsy, and confirms the importance of detecting clinically occult (microscopic) metastases as a predictor of survival. In the approximately 16% of patients who had nodal metastases, they were detected a median of 16 months earlier in the group having a sentinel node biopsy compared to the "watch and wait" approach. In the SLN biopsy arm, SLN status was the most significant predictor of survival in a multifactorial analysis. These results confirm other analyses specifically examining the prognostic significance of SLN biopsy.

The use of sentinel lymph node biopsy offers significant benefits. It provides excellent prognostic information; patients with node negative disease can be accurately classified as low-risk patients without a complete node dissection. Patients with a positive sentinel node biopsy can undergo a completion dissection and be considered for adjuvant therapy or clinical trials if deemed appropriate. Numerous large studies of patients undergoing sentinel node biopsy show that regional control of the targeted node basin is excellent both in the node positive and node negative groups. The routine use of sentinel node biopsy as a staging tool allows for more accurate stratification of patients entering trials of adjuvant systemic therapies. The concept of the sentinel node is now well established and should be used in all melanoma patients where the staging information will be useful for staging and treatment planning.

Rationale for Surgical Treatment Options

Every primary melanoma requires a wide excision for local control. The size of the surgical margin must be tailored to the tumor thickness and the anatomic location of the melanoma. Decades ago, all melanomas were excised with a 4–5 cm margin. A series of prospective, randomized surgical trials have clearly shown that a reduced surgical excision is safe and appropriate for all primary melanomas. The World Health Organization Melanoma Programme randomized

612 patients with primary melanoma less than 2 mm in thickness to be treated with either 1 cm or 3 cm margins. The two randomized groups did not differ significantly in either local recurrence rate or in 10-year survival rate. Thus a 1 cm margin is recognized as appropriate margin for all T1 (1 mm) melanomas and for many T2 (1.01–2.0 mm) melanomas.

The Intergroup Melanoma Surgical Trial randomized 740 patients with intermediate thickness melanomas (1.0–4.0 mm) to determine whether a 2 cm radial margin of excision is equivalent to a 4 cm radial margin with respect to survival and local recurrence rates. Patients with melanomas located on a trunk or proximal extremity(N = 468) were randomized to receive either a 2 or 4 cm excision margin. Patients assigned to 2 cm margin were much less likely to require a skin graft and experienced no diminution in overall survival or local recurrence rates compared to patients who had a 4 cm surgical excision. Ulceration of the primary lesion was found to be associated with a dramatic increase in local recurrence rates. Among all the patients randomized, the local recurrence rates were 6.6% for all ulcerated melanomas versus 1.1% for all non-ulcerated melanomas.

Thomas and colleagues reported the results of a randomized controlled trial in the United Kingdom in which patients with melanomas thicker than 2 mm were randomized to resection with either 1 cm or 3 cm margins. No surgical intervention of the regional node basin was allowed. In the trial, 453 patients had excision with a 1 cm margin of excision and 447 with a 3 cm margin. There were 168 loco-regional recurrences in the patients with 1 cm compared with 142 in the group with 3 cm margins (Hazard ratio, 1.26; 95% confidence interval, 1–1.59; P = 0.05); most of the recurrences in each group were nodal rather than local. Thus, the patients with 1 cm margins had a significantly increased risk of loco-regional recurrence compared to those with 3 cm margins; however, overall survival was equivalent in the two groups.

When considering the results of the Intergroup Surgical Melanoma Trial and the UK study together, wide excision with 2 cm margin is appropriate management for intermediate thickness melanoma(T2 and T3). No randomized studies have been done specifically targeted at appropriate margins for T4 (>4 mm) melanomas. A retrospective study at The University of Texas M.D. Anderson Cancer Center showed no difference in local recurrence rates or survival in patients with T4 melanoma who received a <2 cm margin compared to those who underwent excision with >2 cm radial margin. Thus there appears to be no advantage in margins wider than 2 cm for patients with thick melanoma. Figure 10.2 displays a decision tree for surgical management of Stage I and II melanoma.

Patients with resectable regional disease (positive regional nodes or limited in transit lesions) should undergo surgical resection for regional control and possible cure. Those with positive nodes should have a formal, anatomic lymphadenectomy as the standard of care. Quantification of the value of complete lymphadenectomy in patients with positive nodes is under evaluation in randomized clinical trials. Limited in transit lesions should be excised to a negative margin. For patients with Stage IV disease, surgery is usually limited to

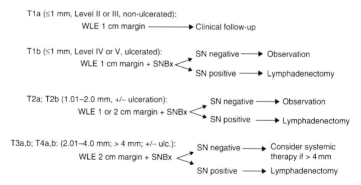

FIGURE 10.2. Surgical management of clinical Stage I and II melanoma. Note: SN = sentinel node, SNBx = lymphatic mapping and sentinel node biopsy, WLE = wide local excision. Sentinel nodes should be evaluated with multiple levels and immunohistochemical staining. All patients with positive nodes or melanoma > 4 mm should be strongly considered for interferon or a clinical trial of systemic adjuvant therapy.

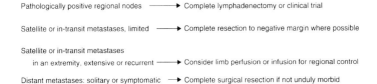

FIGURE 10.3. Surgical management of Stage III and IV melanoma. Note: All Stage III and IV patients should be strongly considered for systemic therapy. Clinical trials are encouraged. Radiation therapy should be considered after lymphadenectomy for patients with >4 positive nodes or extranodal extension.

palliation of specific, symptomatic lesions, although there are rare reports in the literature of prolonged survival following resection of solitary metastatic lesions. Clinical trials of systemic therapy are encouraged for patients with Stage III and Stage IV disease. Figure 10.3 displays a decision tree for the management of Stage III and IV melanoma.

Follow-Up

The risk of recurrence for patients with surgically treated melanoma is related to pathologic features of the melanoma at its presentation, especially the tumor thickness, the presence of ulceration, and the presence of nodal metastases. Common sites of locoregional recurrence are near the primary excision site and the regional nodal basin. Common sites of distant recurrences include cutaneous and subcutaneous sites distant from the primary, distant lymph nodes, and the lungs. Less commonly, first relapses may involve the liver, brain or bone. Melanoma can have an unpredictable metastatic pattern and can spread to unusual sites such as the gastrointestinal tract.

For most patients with surgically treated Stage I, II, or III disease, recommended follow-up is primarily with periodic history and physical exam. Routine radiologic tests and screening blood tests have not been documented to improve survival, but may be considered at the discretion of the treating physician. While most recurrences will occur within the first 2 to 3 years after diagnosis, late recurrences (even after 10 years) can occur. There is no clear evidence that structured follow-up of patients with treated melanoma will change outcome. However, routine surveillance may allow earlier detection of disease recurrence, when it is more likely to be surgically resectable, and will keep the patient in contact with medical providers.

Selected Readings

Balch CM, Buzaid AC, Atkins MB, et al. (2001) Final Version of the American Joint Committee on Cancer Staging System for Cutaneous Melanoma. J Clin Oncol 19:3635–3648

Balch CM, Houghton AN, Sober AJ, Soong S (1998) Cutaneous melanoma. Quality Medical Publishing, St. Louis, MO

Balch CM, Soong S (2000) Long-term results of a multi-institutional randomized trial comparing prognostic factors and surgical results for intermediate thickness melanomas (1.0 to 4.0 mm). Intergroup Melanoma Surgical Trial. Ann Surg Oncol 7: 87–97

Balch CM, Soong SJ, Gershenwald JE, et al. (2001) Prognostic factors analysis of 17,600 melanoma patients: validation of the American Joint Committee on Cancer melanoma staging system. J Clin Oncol 19:3622–3634

Gershenwald JE, Thompson W, Mansfield PF, et al. (1999) Multi-institutional melanoma lymphatic mapping experience: the prognostic value of sentinel lymph node status in 612 stageI or II melanoma patients. JClin Oncol 17:976–983

Gimotty PA, Botbyl J, Soong SJ, Guerry D (2005) A population-based validation of the AJCC melanoma staging system. J Clin Oncol 23:8065

Morton DL, Thompson JF, Cochran AJ, et al. (2006) Sentinel node biopsy compared to nodal observation in melanoma. N Engl J Med 355:1307–1317

Morton D, Wen D, Wong J, et al. (1992) Technical details of intraoperative lymphatic mapping for early stage melanoma. Arch Surg 127:392–399

Veronesi U, Cascinelli N (1991) Narrow excision (1-cm margin). A safe procedure for thin cutaneous melanoma, Arch Surg 126:438–441

11
Technique and Application of Sentinel Lymph Node Biopsy in Melanoma

Marshall M. Urist

Pearls and Pitfalls

- Apply the histological parameters of the melanoma and the physical findings to determine the probability of finding a positive sentinel lymph node (SLN).
- Examine the patient carefully for scars because previous surgical procedures may alter lymphatic pathways and ensure valid lymphatic mapping.
- Discuss the location of common and aberrant nodal sites with the patient prior to the mapping procedure.
- Injection of the radioisotope should be only at the intra-dermal level. Subcutaneous injections may dissect along tissue planes and obscure SLNs.
- Observe the radioisotope scan early after injection (especially in the head and neck area) and be observant for aberrant pathways.
- On the trunk and extremities, SLN biopsy can be performed as a separate procedure after wide local excision (WLE); however, injections around the scar can drain to more nodes than would have been involved before WLE.
- Palpate the wound cavity after removal of the SLN to detect unseen nodes replaced by metastatic melanoma.

K.I. Bland et al. (eds.), *Surgery in Breast Cancer and Melanoma*, DOI 10.1007/978-1-84996-435-7_11, © Springer-Verlag London Limited 2011

Introduction

Lymphatic mapping with SLN biopsy is the most significant advance in the surgical treatment of melanoma in the last 30 years. Successful application of this method requires close collaboration between surgeons, pathologists, and radiologists. With qualified instruction, the technique can be learned and mastered in a few months. Interim results from ongoing prospective trials have shown that SLN biopsy increases the accuracy of staging, provides important prognostic information, and may prolong survival in patients with subclinical metastases.

Basic Science

Lymphoscintigraphy was developed in the 1970s to identify the draining nodal basin in patients with melanoma who were being considered for elective (prophylactic) lymph node dissections. Two decades later, Dr. Donald Morton and colleagues developed and tested the concept of the SLN. In theory, a label (radioisotope or visible dye) injected into the skin at the primary site will travel through the same lymphatic pathway taken by tumor cells in reaching a regional lymph node. This node, the SLN, should be the first to contain metastatic tumor cells if any are present. This principle has been confirmed in many publications which show that the technique is more accurate in identifying metastases and is associated with fewer side effects than complete axillary lymph node dissection.

Lymphatic anatomy has been studied extensively and shown to be frequently predictable, although variability in lymphatic flow may be evident. The midline defines the side to which lymphatics drain; however, sites within 2–3 cm of the midline can drain bilaterally or to the contralateral side alone. Transversely, Sappey's line defines a band of skin extending from the umbilicus, along the iliac crests over to L1. This line divides sites which drain to the axilla above, the groin below, or both sites. Popliteal and epitrochlear nodes receive direct drainage from relatively small areas of skin on the leg and forearm, respectively. Sites on the scalp, neck, and face frequently drain in multiple directions. Lymphoscintigraphy regularly highlights nodal sites outside the expected basins in all anatomic areas.

While mapping techniques often identify a single node, there are many instances wherein the drainage is to multiple nodes. Mapped nodes should be removed and analyzed when blue or containing sufficient levels of radioactivity (see below).

Clinical Presentation and Patient Selection

The consensus-based treatment guidelines from the National Comprehensive Cancer Network (NCCN) summarize recommendations for all aspects of melanoma patient care (Fig. 11.1). Patients being considered for SLN biopsy have a confirmed diagnosis of invasive melanoma. These patients should undergo a complete history focused on previously diagnosed skin lesions and the family history. The physical examination should include a complete examination of the skin, lymphatic basins, and potential sites of metastasis. Laboratory and radiologic evaluations have a very low probability of showing metastatic disease in asymptomatic patients. These staging studies should be reserved for symptomatic patients or those with locally advanced tumors and/or adenopathy.

The decision to perform an SLN biopsy begins with a complete pathological analysis of the primary tumor. The following parameters should be defined in the pathology report in cases of invasive melanoma: Breslow thickness, Clark's level, ulceration, growth pattern, regression, lymphocytic infiltration, and mitotic index. The risk of spread of melanoma to a regional node increases with tumor thickness. Unfortunately, there is not a well-defined thickness at which there is no risk of metastasis. It is now generally accepted that the risk begins to be significant when the tumor cells have penetrated to a depth of 1 mm. The risk can be altered by other factors including ulceration, regression, age, and site. A useful nomogram has

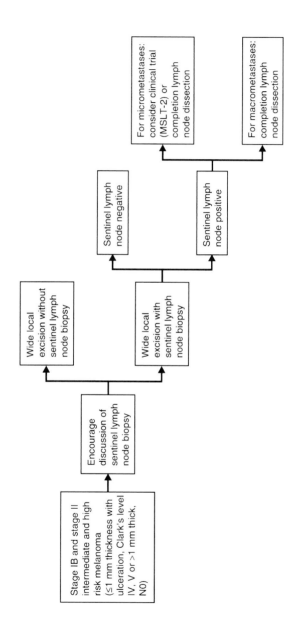

FIGURE 11.1. Algorithm for the management of regional lymph nodes in patients with cutaneous melanoma (based on guidelines from the National Comprehensive Cancer Network).

been developed to define the probability of finding a positive sentinel node and it is available on the NCCN website. The presence of ulceration, regression, and/or extension of the melanoma to Clark's level IV or V have been used as indications for SLN biopsy for tumors measuring <1 mm in thickness. More outcome studies will need to be performed to reach consensus on this point.

Over 30 years ago it was shown that the detailed analysis of lymph nodes could increase the detection rate of metastases from breast cancer. This process requires serial sections from each node and is not practical when the specimen includes a large number of nodes. The advantage of the SLN method is that the pathologist can focus attention on a relatively low number of nodes and maximize the detection rate. Lymph nodes are serially sectioned at 1–2 mm intervals. Nodes are first analyzed using standard H&E staining. When metastases are not seen by H&E, immunohistochemistry techniques using S-100, HMB-45, and other antigenic markers are utilized.

The prognosis for melanoma patients is related to the number of involved regional nodes. The TNM staging system for melanoma has been altered to define the size of the metastasis in regional nodes. Clinically occult (microscopic) metastases are classified as N1a (one positive node) and N2a (2–3 positive nodes). Clinically apparent macroscopic metastases are classified as N1b (one positive node) or N2b (2–3 positive nodes). Patients with microscopic nodal metastases have a significantly better prognosis than those with macroscopic metastases.

Treatment/Technique

Informed Consent

At the present time SLN biopsy is a valuable staging procedure, therefore, discussions with the patient must emphasize both the value and limitations of the technique. Since melanoma can be a lethal disease, there is great value in understanding the true prognosis. When the sentinel node is negative, it will not only reassure the patient that the prognosis is favorable, but also define a less intensive follow-up schedule. When the node is positive, the patient should be counseled about prognosis, staging procedures, follow-up examinations, and protocols for adjuvant therapy. It is important for the patient to understand that performance of the SLN biopsy has shown a survival advantage only for lymph node-positive patients. See outcomes below.

Operative Procedure

The lymphoscintigram is performed by injecting 0.05 mCi of 99mTc sulfur colloid intradermally around the primary tumor or biopsy site. Larger diameter tumors or long biopsy incisions require injection at intervals around the entire area. Injection into the subcutaneous space should be avoided because this can dissect along tissue planes and obscure detection of nearby nodes. In most cases the sentinel node will appear within 15 min. It is important to observe the scanner from the time of injection because multiple nodes may appear and the sequence of their appearance will not necessarily be in the order of the distance from the injection site. Tissues in the head and neck area are richly supplied with lymphatics which can both facilitate and complicate the process. If the SLN is very close to the primary site, detection can be masked by the injection site radioactivity. It is important to observe the patient under the scanner early in the procedure. The lymphoscintigram may show multiple lymphatic channels leading to the same node (Fig. 11.2).

When the patient returns to the operating room, the position of the radioactive node(s) is confirmed with a hand-held gamma detection probe before the patient is prepped and draped for the operation. The location may be somewhat different than the site as mapped from the lymphoscintigram.

The second phase of the operative procedure is the injection of a visible blue dye, isosulfan blue (Lymphazurin 1%,

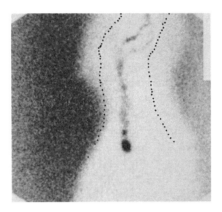

FIGURE 11.2. Lymphoscintigram: left lateral view with the patient's arm extended over the head. Note two lymphatic vessels draining from the forearm to the same axillary sentinel lymph node (SLN).

Ben Venue Labs) at the primary tumor biopsy site. This is an intradermal injection of 0.5–1.0 ml of dye in 3–6 sites around the biopsy or scar. Subcutaneous injection of blue dye should be avoided because it can dissect along tissue planes and obscure the surgeon's view of the node. If the node is very close to the primary site, a lower volume of dye will allow identification of the node without forcing dye into the interstitial space.

The incision is placed close to the radioactive site to allow minimal dissection to obtain the node. The scar should be oriented to allow it to be incorporated into the line of a completion lymph node dissection (CLND) if this becomes necessary. Once the skin is open, the dissection is carried along the tract toward the radioactive source. Blue lymphatic channels are often seen as the dissection approaches the node. Multiple nodes may be involved. All blue or radioactive nodes are removed. In most patients there are 1–3 sentinel nodes in a single basin. When each node is removed, it is counted with the gamma probe and labeled. By convention, the procedure is considered complete when the count in the bed of the resected node(s) is <10% of the highest ex vivo sentinel node count. When all blue and radioactive nodes are removed, the wound is palpated to detect any firm or enlarged nodes. Tumor obliterating a node might block the flow of lymph and prevent the uptake of dye or isotope. Nodes detected in this manner are also counted as sentinel nodes.

In some instances, the SLN will be very close to the primary site and not detectable on the lymphoscintigram. Blocking the injection site may reveal the node on the scan. In other circumstances, the node can only be detected after resection of the primary site and reapplication of the gamma probe. When the primary site is not in proximity to the nodal basin and the SLN does not appear on the lymphoscintigram, the scan should be repeated at another time.

Additional surgical considerations apply for specific sites. In the groin, the incision is placed directly over the radioactive node. The skin in the axilla is more mobile, therefore, the incision is placed over a skin fold at the lower edge of the hair-bearing area. The neck incisions may need to be moved closer to the line of a future neck dissection incision. Using primarily blunt dissection, nodes in the area of the parotid can be safely removed because most sentinel nodes are immediately under the capsule of the parotid gland. If the node is deeper, further dissection will incur a higher risk of facial nerve injury.

Outcome

A well-accepted tenant of cancer treatment states that earlier diagnosis leads to an improved outcome. The corollary, earlier diagnosis of regional metastatic disease leads to improved outcome, is not uniformly accepted. This hypothesis is being tested in the Multi-institutional Selective Lymphadenectomy Trial 1 (MSLT-1) in which patients with intermediate thickness melanoma (1.2–3.5 mm) undergoing WLE were randomly assigned to observation (500 patients) or SLN biopsy (764 patients). Earlier reports from the MSLT-1 confirmed that the technique was safe and associated with a low morbidity rate.

The accuracy of the technique continued to improve as centers extended their experience. After a median follow-up of 59.8 months (third of five planned analyses), there was no difference in overall survival or melanoma-specific survival between the two groups. This is not surprising, as only 16% of patients had a positive SLN and, therefore, could have potentially benefited from the operation. Interestingly, exactly the same percentage of patients were diagnosed with regional nodal metastases in both groups, suggesting that even micrometastases have the potential to develop into clinically detectable metastases. There was a higher number of tumor-bearing lymph nodes in the delayed group compared to the SLN group, 3.3 nodes vs. 1.4 nodes, $p = < 0.001$, respectively. Survival rates for the lymph node-positive patients did show a significant difference in favor of SLN biopsy compared to observation, $72.3 \pm 4.6\%$ vs. $52.4 \pm 5.9\%$, $p = 0.004$. Thus far in this important study, SLN biopsy provided accurate prognostic information and improved the survival in patients with positive nodes when compared with those undergoing delayed lymph node dissection.

When a SLN was positive, patients underwent CLND. Experience in this trial and previous nonrandomized reports has shown that <10% of lymph node basins will harbor additional positive nodes. Because of this low probability of benefit, the MSLT Group has launched a second trial to randomize node-positive patients to CLND versus observation with delayed dissection if further nodes are detected. This observation schedule includes high-resolution ultrasound examinations, which have been shown to reliably detect metastases 5 mm in diameter.

The SLN concept and technique were rapidly learned and accepted by the surgical community worldwide. It is now considered to be a standard technique in melanoma patient care based upon the valuable diagnostic information it provides. Patients are greatly relieved by the good news of a negative sentinel node. On the other hand, patients with a positive sentinel node have the opportunity to undergo appropriate staging studies and learn about clinical trials for adjuvant therapy.

Selected Readings

Balch CM, Soong S-J, Gershenwald JE, et al. (2001) Prognostic factors analysis of 17,600 melanoma patients: Validation of the American Joint Committee on Cancer Melanoma Staging System. J Clin Oncol 19:3622–3634

Houghton AN, Coit DG, Daud A, et al. (2006) Melanoma. J Natl Comp Canc Netw 7:666–684. National Comprehensive Cancer Network Guidelines for the Management of Melanoma are revised annually and are available online at www.nccn.org

Morton DL, Cochran AJ, Thompson JF, et al. (2005). Sentinel node biopsy for early-stage melanoma accuracy and morbidity in MSLT-1, an International Multicenter Trial. Ann Surg 242:302–313

Morton DL, Thompson JF, Cochran AJ, et al. (2006) Sentinel-node biopsy or nodal observation in melanoma. N Engl J Med 355:1307–1317

Morton DL, Wen DR, Wong JH, et al. (1992) Technical details of intra-operative lymphatic mapping for early stage melanoma. Arch Surg 127:392–399

Pincon AI, Coit DG, Shaha AR, et al. (2006) Sentinel lymph node biopsy for cutaneous head and neck melanoma: Mapping the parotid gland. Ann Surg Oncol (published online May, 2006)

Starritt EC, Uren RF, Scolyer RA, et al. (2005) Ultrasound examination of sentinel nodes in the initial assessment of patients with primary cutaneous melanoma. Ann Surg Oncol 12:18–23

Wong SL, Kattan W, McMasters KM, Coit DG (2005) A nomogram that predicts the presence of sentinel node metastasis in melanoma with better discrimination than the American Joint Committee on Cancer staging system. Ann Surg Oncol 12:282–288

12
Surgical Treatment of Malignant Melanoma

Stanley P.L. Leong

Pearls and Pitfalls

- Any changes in a skin lesion should be suspicious of a melanoma.
- Microstaging is the most important information for the extent of the excision for primary melanoma.
- Melanoma is progressive, therefore, earlier diagnosis and excision is the key for a potential cure.
- Selective sentinel lymphadenectomy (SSL) has replaced elective lymph node dissection as a standard of care for staging the regional nodal basin with primary melanoma of equal or greater than 1 mm.
- SSL is a multidisciplinary procedure involving the support of nuclear medicine for preoperative lymphoscintigraphy, expertise to be developed by surgeons intraoperatively and careful examination of the sentinel lymph nodes postoperatively by pathologists. Preoperative lymphoscintigraphy is mandatory for defining the draining nodal basins including in-transit, epitrochlear, and popliteal sites.
- Stage III melanoma with grossly palpable disease should be aggressively treated with radical lymph node dissection.
- Isolated (solitary) metastatic melanoma should be resected if possible.
- Melanoma should be approached in a multidisciplinary fashion. Therefore, it is not prudent to render treatment decision alone but should solicit multidisciplinary consensus.

K.I. Bland et al. (eds.), *Surgery in Breast Cancer and Melanoma*, DOI 10.1007/978-1-84996-435-7_12,
© Springer-Verlag London Limited 2011

- Melanoma may occur in different anatomical sites, therefore, in certain surgical sites beyond the surgical breadths of the surgeon, consultant surgeon should be invited to participate in surgery.
- Although SSL appears to be a minimally invasive procedure, expertise needs to be developed in the head and neck area particularly in the parotid region where the facial nerves should be carefully mapped out with a nerve stimulator, adequate exposure should be available for axillary lymph nodes from the deep axillary area close to the axillary vein from a relatively small opening, potential separate sentinel lymph nodes may be present in the superficial inguinal (femoral) or deep inguinal (external iliac) basin. The surgeon should be familiar with the complicated anatomy of all the nodal basins.
- Be aware of anaphylactic reaction to blue dye during intra-operative lymphatic mapping.
- Any symptoms for a patient with melanoma should be suspected of potential reoccurrence and, therefore, appropriate work up should be pursued to rule out metastatic melanoma.

Introduction

The incidence of melanoma has increased significantly over the past 35 years and is currently about 1 of 70 Americans, mainly Caucasians. About 62,000 melanoma patients are diagnosed and over 7,000 patients die of the disease annually. Whether increasing melanoma incidence is real or due to improved diagnosis still needs to be determined. Despite the incidence doubling every 10 years, the overall mortality from melanoma has increased only slightly. This trend suggests that a significant proportion of the melanoma being diagnosed is of the thin level and can be effectively treated by definitive surgical resection. Surgical treatment of primary invasive melanoma has become more individualized, based on microstaging information of primary melanoma and the sentinel lymph node status of the regional nodal basin. This chapter addresses the issues a surgeon will face in dealing with a patient with a newly-diagnosed or recurrent melanoma.

Diagnosis of Melanoma and Initial Evaluation

When a cutaneous lesion or mole undergoes a change in size, color, shape, contour or sensation, it should be biopsied. An excisional biopsy of 2 mm margin is usually done so that the entire lesion, including the subcutaneous fat, can be submitted to the pathologist for histologic diagnosis and microstaging. The primary reason for an excisional biopsy is twofold: (1) although an incisional biopsy may establish the diagnosis of melanoma, a subsequent completion biopsy is necessary to determine the thickness of melanoma; and (2) a small specimen will sometimes make identifying the diagnosis difficult, especially in acral lentiginous and lentigo malignant melanomas. For these reasons, a shave biopsy should be abandoned because shaving the entire level of the melanoma will compromise subsequent level and thickness determination. In general, if the lesion is smaller than 2 cm in diameter, it should be completely excised, with a 2 mm margin. However, if the lesion is larger than 2 cm or if it is at a site such as the face or digit that does not lend itself to excisional biopsy, an incisional biopsy of the most suspicious area using a scalpel or a skin punch is a reasonable approach. Patients with pigmented lesions often see a dermatologist, who frequently does the initial biopsy of a suspected mole. When the diagnosis is established, the patient will be referred to a surgeon for definitive surgical treatment. Therefore, surgeons must interact closely with their dermatologist colleagues so that the sequence of events can be traced to the time of biopsy. In this respect, surgeons also work very closely with pathologists to obtain the diagnosis and microstaging of melanoma for surgical treatment. When a melanoma is diagnosed, the initial evaluation of the patient should include a complete history with emphasis on occupational or environmental exposure to sunlight, as well as any accompanying conditions that might compromise immunity. In addition, a family history should be taken, as about 10% of melanomas have a strong familial linkage. A thorough physical examination, including a total body skin examination and palpation of the regional lymph nodes is important. The emphasis of this evaluation is to identify risk factors, signs or symptoms of metastases, atypical moles and synchronous melanomas.

The initial laboratory evaluation consists of CBC, blood chemistries for renal and hepatic functions, and chest x-ray. For thin melanoma (<1 mm thickness), extensive diagnostic studies such as computed axial tomography (CT), magnetic resonance imaging (MRI) and nuclear scans, are not indicated and should not be used to stage these patients. However, for thicker melanoma, or if there is suspicion that the patient has metastatic disease associated with symptoms, appropriate scans should be done.

In general, when melanoma is diagnosed early and is less than 1 mm thick, the cure rate approaches over 95%. If melanoma is not detected until the thickness becomes over 4 mm, the survival rate drops to less than 50%. Early diagnosis has been achieved by education, screening and digital dermatoscopy, which can monitor suspicious pigmented lesions serially so that they can be removed earlier for any changes based on the digital pictures recorded in the computer system.

Staging of Melanoma

It is important to microstage melanoma with Clark's levels (I–IV), categorizing the tumor by the level of invasion into the dermal layers of the skin and subcutaneous fat, and Breslow's tumor depth, measuring thickness of the lesion from top to bottom, to guide the extent of re-excision. A melanoma staging system should include all manifestations of the disease with biologic predictive value, but at the same time, must be simple enough to be adopted universally. Pursuit of this goal prompted the American Joint Committee on Cancer (AJCC) and Union Internationale Centre le Cancer (UICC) to jointly propose a single pTNM (primary tumor, nodes and metastases) staging system for cutaneous melanoma. Recent AJCC clarification has resulted in the universal adoption of this system, which also includes the sentinel lymph node (SLN) status.

Surgical Treatment of Stage 1 Melanoma

The surgeon must know the exact original size of the melanoma to reconstruct it within the context of the biopsy scar. The center of the scar can be used as a reference point by which exact measurement can be derived in order to include it within the resection margin. In general, the scar is thought to be potentially contaminated by microscopic tumor cells from previous biopsy, although, no conclusive data is available to demonstrate this. The rationale for wide excision of melanoma is based on the fact that complete removal of microscopic melanoma cells situated adjacent to the primary melanoma may result in decreased local recurrence and subsequent metastasis. Most major melanoma treatment centers agree that excision margins can be tailored to the thickness of melanoma (Table 12.1). Excision of the fascia is optional. In areas with deep subcutaneous tissue, it is probably not necessary to excise the fascia. On the other hand, when the melanoma is thick and the subcutaneous tissue is relatively thin, the fascia may be excised to obtain a more adequate deep margin. When the fascia is aponeurosis of the muscle, the aponeurosis should be spared. Three approaches

TABLE 12.1. Surgical excision margins for primary melanoma according to National Comprehensive Cancer Network guidelines (Houghton et al., 2006).

Melanoma in situ	Margin[a] (cm)
Thickness of invasive melanoma (mm)	
≤1	1
1.01–2.00	1–2
2.01–4.00	2
>4	2

[a] Margins may be changed to adjust to individual anatomic or cosmetic considerations.

may be used to close the surgical defect: (1) a primary closure, (2) a split-thickness skin graft, and (3) a full-thickness flap. In general, primary closure should be the goal in most anatomical sites as it is preferable for cosmetic and psychological reasons. In most cases, rotational flaps are not required. Melanoma sites such as the face, ear, breast, digits, hands, feet, penis, mucosa and the retina deserve special attention. For more detailed information, please see additional references.

Local and In-Transit Recurrent Melanoma

For practical purposes, it is important to define local recurrence in terms of persistent disease, which is defined as locally recurrent disease that is usually in a scar, with junctional melanocytic proliferation. It is biologically different from recurrent melanoma in dermis and also cutaneous fat, for example, as a microsatellite or in-transit metastasis. Persistent disease is not, in general, a reflection of aggressive biological behavior, but rather inadequate surgical margins. Recurrent disease may occur with adequate margins and reflects more aggressive biologic behavior. Microsatellites are sometimes found in sections of the primary site in tumors thicker than 2 mm. They appear to be more common than clinical satellitosis, but both are associated with a poorer prognosis. In addition, a local recurrence is associated with a high mortality rate of about 60–80%. A local recurrence can be excised usually with a 1 cm radius margin using primary closure. Isolated in-transit metastatic melanoma may be excised locally. More extensive in-transit metastases in the extremities may be treated by heated isolated limb perfusion. However, adjuvant limb perfusion is not recommended.

Selective Sentinel Lymphadenectomy for Melanoma

Selective sentinel lymphadenectomy (SSL) should be considered standard of care for staging patients with primary invasive melanoma 1 mm or greater. To minimize the false-negative rate, surgeons, nuclear medicine physicians, and pathologists should work as a multidisciplinary team to achieve the best result for the patient. Steps for SSL consist of the following: (1) preoperative lymphoscintigraphy, (2) injection of radio-isotope, (3) identification of lymphatic basins, (4) determining type of anesthesia (local or general), (5) intraoperative mapping technique, (6) injection of isosulfan blue dye, (7) intraoperative mapping with a handheld gamma probe, (8) identification of sentinel lymph nodes (SLNs), and (9) pathologic examination of SLNs by hematoxylin and eosin staining and immunohistochemistry. Figure 12.1 shows the algorithm for treating a patient with melanoma ≥1 mm. When the SLNs are negative, the patient may be monitored without having to undergo a complete regional lymph node dissection. For more detailed information in SSL with respect to different nodal basins (see Leong, 2005).

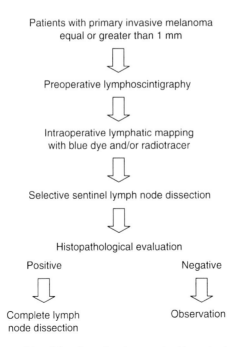

Patients with primary invasive melanoma
equal or greater than 1 mm

Preoperative lymphoscintigraphy

Intraoperative lymphatic mapping
with blue dye and/or radiotracer

Selective sentinel lymph node dissection

Histopathological evaluation

Positive   Negative

Complete lymph   Observation
node dissection

FIGURE 12.1. Algorithm for selective sentinel lymphadenectomy.

A SLN may be blue, hot, or any lymph node greater than 10% of the in vivo count of the hottest lymph node. An enlarged or indurated lymph node should be removed because it may contain metastatic cancer cells that block blue dye or radiotracer entry. Surgeons who use isosulfan blue dye should be cognizant of treatment for a potentially fatal reaction. Prophylactic lymph node dissection should not be performed if a SSL can be performed as a staging procedure. A complete lymph node dissection is performed if the SLN is positive. The role of SSL is to provide accurate staging at the initial diagnosis of primary invasive melanoma ≥ 1 mm because the staging result is often accurate, the morbidity is reduced, and the cost is less.

Tanis et al. [5] recently studied the effect of frozen section investigation of the SLN in malignant melanoma. Analysis of frozen sections showed metastasis in 8 of 17 patients with node-positive melanoma out of a group of 99 melanoma patients. The sensitivity was 41% and the specificity was 100%. The authors concluded that frozen section analyses is not recommended for patients with melanoma. False negative results from SSL may result from the following: (1) failed preoperative lymphoscintigraphy, including injection techniques; (2) interpretation of the lymphoscintigraphy; (3) failed intraoperative lymphatic mapping; (4) failed pathological evaluation; (5) skip metastasis; and (6) too few cells only detectable by polymerase chain reaction analysis. In general, the 10% rule by McMasters et al. seems to be a reasonable guide that suggests all blue lymph nodes and all nodes that measure 10% or higher of the ex vivo radioactive count of the hottest sentinel node should be excised.

Surgical Treatment for Stage III Disease with Nodal Basin Involvement

When a regional lymph node is involved, the 5-year survival rate ranges from 30% to 60%, depending on the tumor burden in the lymph node(s) and the number of lymph nodes involved.

The survival rate drops to single digits when metastasis is found beyond the regional lymph nodes, especially in visceral sites. In the past, the only way to detect metastasis in the regional lymph nodes was to do a complete or radical lymph node dissection, which might be associated with increased morbidity such as lymphedema. The most important development since 1992 is the demonstration that the regional nodal basin may be best assessed by selectively removing the SLN, as it is the first lymph node in the regional nodal basin to receive the cancer cells from the primary site. Therefore, at the initial diagnosis of the primary melanoma, it is quite reliable to assess the regional nodal basin by selectively taking out one or a few SLNs to determine whether there are any cancer cells in these lymph nodes, as mentioned above. If they are negative, the chance of having additional cancer cells in the nodal basin is less than 5%. Thus, over 80% of the patients may be spared a more extensive and morbid radical lymph node dissection after a negative SLN is removed.

Therapeutic Lymph Node Dissection

Since surgery may achieve a 25–30% overall control rate for stage III disease and over 85% for regional nodal control, and no systemic treatment is available, an adequate lymph node dissection to resect the metastatic melanoma is crucial to achieve both excellent local control and potential long-term control. In general, the entire regional lymph node content should be removed en bloc, along with the enlarged lymph nodes, in a procedure known as a radical regional lymph node dissection. The procedure entails a radical axillary lymph node dissection including level I, II, and III; a radical ilioinguinal lymph node dissection for possible pelvic lymph node involvement and a modified radical neck dissection with ipsilateral involvement. Care should be taken not to enter the tumor, which could significantly increase the recurrence rate in the regional area. If multiple lymph nodes are involved or disease extends beyond the capsule, postoperative adjuvant radiation therapy may be considered.

Resection of Metastatic Melanoma

Patients with recurrence tend to have them at local or regional sites that may be amenable to surgical intervention. Studies have shown that if isolated metastatic melanoma is resectable, such as that in bowel, lung, and liver, it should be resected. Of course, it will be futile to resect multiple visceral sites.

Follow-Up Monitoring of Melanoma Patients

The prognosis for long-term survival for patients with early invasive melanoma (<1 mm) is excellent, over 95% for a 10-year period. Overall, there is about a 3% increase of primary melanomas in affected patients. The risk may be higher in patients with associated atypical moles and is particularly higher (approximately 33%) in affected members of melanoma-prone families. Therefore, these patients need closer follow-up to watch for the development of a second primary melanoma as subsequent melanomas diagnosed in a surveillance program are thinner than the incident melanoma.

Follow-up of stage I patients consists of physical examination, including skin and lymph node sites every 4–6 months. Laboratory testing with CBC, liver function tests and chest X-ray may be required. Although no specific marker is available for melanoma, elevated serum lactate dehydrogenase (LDH) level is a useful marker of metastatic disease. Patients with high-risk melanoma or regional node metastasis should be seen at 3–4 month intervals. Patients with atypical moles should be monitored for second primary melanomas, and the baseline photographs for future comparisons may be useful. Follow-up examination of atypical moles with serial photographs may be carried out by a dermatologist who is interested in the management of early melanoma. Patients can assist in their follow-up care by examining their skin on a monthly basis. In addition, patients with the diagnosis of melanoma should be encouraged to avoid excessive sun exposure and to use protective clothing and sunscreens with an SPF of at least 15. Patients with atypical moles or a positive family history should be enrolled along with their family members into a regular screening program, which may be supervised by an experienced dermatologist. In general, melanoma patients should be followed for earlier detection of reoccurrences, providing reassurance to patients and educating patients for self examination. Despite the fact that the prognosis of thin melanoma (<1 mm thick) is excellent, a few may recur over a long period of time. Therefore even patients with thin melanomas should undergo lifelong follow-up monitoring.

Complications

Complications from radical neck, axillary, and inguinal lymph node dissection have been previously described. Therefore, only complications of SSL will be discussed further here. They consist of seroma, wound infection, sensory loss and lymphedema associated with SSL for melanoma in the axilla and groin. One study detailed major (5%) and minor (31%) complications from SSL for melanoma in 100 consecutive patients. We have recently conducted a prospective analysis of complications for melanoma patients undergoing SSL in which we collected follow-up data on post-operative SSL melanoma patients to evaluate complications. The subject population consisted of patients with invasive melanoma ≥1 mm, who underwent wide local re-excision and SSL between February 2003 and September 2004 at UCSF Comprehensive Cancer Center. Of the 99 patients included, 44 had melanoma on the upper extremity, 31 on the trunk and 24 on the lower extremity. The initial post-operative complications from the primary melanoma excision sites were numbness (47.5%), pain (16.2%), cellulitis (6.1%), and wound separation (3%). For the SSL sites (123 SSL procedures performed), complications consisted of numbness (37.4%), seroma (24.4%), limb motion restriction (16.3%), pain (15.4%), lymphedema (12.5%), and cellulitis (4.9%). Thirty four patients were followed for 1 year postoperatively (14 upper extremity, 9 trunk, 11 lower extremity). In comparison to primary site complications at the initial post-operative visit, by 1 year after surgery, the numbness rate decreased significantly (11.8%). Pain, cellulitis, and wound separation were no longer present. For the 38 SSL sites followed for 1 year post-operatively, numbness decreased significantly (13.2%), as did lymphedema (8.8%). Pain, limb motion restriction, seroma and cellulitis were no longer present. No patients were hospitalized for any severe complications.

We and others have reported severe anaphylactic reactions from blue dye. In our series, the incidence of anaphylaxis to isosulfan blue was about 0.7%, whereas in others, the incidence ranges from 0.09% to 1.5%. Anaphylaxis can be fatal if not recognized and treated rapidly. Other adverse reactions may include rash or hives.

Selected Readings

Awe WC, Fletcher WS, Krippaehne WW (1965) Incapacitating lymphedema following radical inguinal lymphadenectomy and ipsilateral transverse abdominal incision. Cancer 18:1251–1254

Balch CM et al. (2001) Final version of the American Joint Committee on Cancer staging system for cutaneous melanoma. J Clin Oncol 19: 3635–3648

Hettiaratchy SP et al. (2000) Sentinel lymph node biopsy in malignant melanoma: a series of 100 consecutive patients. Br J Plast Surg 53:559–562

Houghton AN et al. (2006) The NCCN Melanoma Clinical Practice Guidelines in Oncology, version 2

Leong SP, guest ed (2003) Malignant melanoma Part I and II. Surgical Clinics of North America. W.B. Saunders, Philadelphia.

Leong SP (2005) Selective sentinel lymphadenectomy for malignant melanoma, Merkel cell carcinoma, and squamous cell carcinoma. Cancer Treat Res 127:39–76

Leong SP (2004) Sentinel lymph node mapping and selective lymphadenectomy: the standard of care for melanoma. Curr Treat Options Oncol 5:185–194

Morton DL et al. (1992) Technical details of intraoperative lymphatic mapping for early stage melanoma. Arch Surg 127:392–399

Serpell JW, Carne PW, Bailey M (2003) Radical lymph node dissection for melanoma. ANZ J Surg 73:294–299

Starritt EC et al. (2004) Lymphedema after complete axillary node dissection for melanoma: assessment using a new, objective definition. Ann Surg 240:866–874

Tanis PJ et al. (2001) Frozen section investigation of the sentinel node in malignant melanoma and breast cancer. Ann Surg Oncol 8:222–226

13

Surgical and Medical Management of Locally Advanced and Systemic Melanoma

Steven L. Chen, Mark B. Faries, and Donald L. Morton

Pearls and Pitfalls

Primary Cutaneous Melanomas

- The margin of excision should be:1 cm for melanomas ≤ 1mm in thickness; 2 cm for melanomas 1.01–4 mm; and 2–3 cm for melanomas > 4 mm.
- Consider the possibility of re-excision when planning excisional biopsy incisions. In general, extremity excisions should be parallel to the long axis.
- In cosmetically sensitive areas such as the face, or for clinically indistinct lesions such as large in situ melanomas, circumferential punch biopsies can be helpful to confirm that the planned excision margins are negative.

Regional Disease

- Thorough physical examination may reveal palpable nodal disease amenable to fine-needle aspiration, making a sentinel node procedure unnecessary.
- Thin melanomas are unlikely to metastasize in the absence of high-risk factors such as regression or ulceration; an exception is incomplete information on Breslow thickness due to positive deep margins on shave biopsy.

K.I. Bland et al. (eds.), *Surgery in Breast Cancer and Melanoma*, DOI 10.1007/978-1-84996-435-7_13, © Springer-Verlag London Limited 2011

- Sentinel node biopsy is usually indicated to ensure accurate staging and prognosis in patients whose melanomas are thicker than 1 mm.
- Preoperative lymphoscintigraphy can identify efferent flow from primary sites with ambiguous drainage, as well as aberrant drainage to popliteal, epitrochlear, parascapular, or subcostal sentinel nodes.
- Complete lymphadenectomy is usually indicated for any lymphatic basin that contains a tumor-positive sentinel node.

Distant Disease

- Metastasectomy should be undertaken whenever technically feasible, unless tumor doubling time is <40 days.
- Systemic therapies for metastatic disease rarely produce long-term durable responses.
- Radiation therapy can provide significant palliation when surgery is not an option, as for patients with brain and bony metastases.
- Patients should be encouraged to enroll in clinical trials designed to improve therapy outcomes for metastatic melanoma.

Introduction

The incidence of melanoma is increasing at a faster rate than all other malignancies. In the United States, the projected lifetime risk of developing melanoma is 1 in 74 for those born in the year 2000 (Fig. 13.1). Melanoma accounts for approximately 4% of all diagnosed malignancies, and the American Cancer Society estimates that there will be 62,190 melanoma cases this year in the United States. As discussed below, this rapid increase is widely attributed to increased sun and ultraviolet light (UV) exposure.

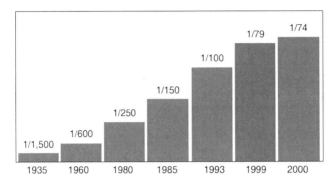

FIGURE 13.1. Lifetime risk of developing invasive melanoma in the United States (Reprinted from Rigel and Carucci, 2000. With permission from Lippincott, Williams & Wilkins).

Risk Factors/Etiology

The primary mechanism for development of sporadic melanoma is thought to be UV-induced damage to DNA in melanocytes (Table 13.1). The higher incidence in fair-complected individuals living in sunnier climes implicates UV exposure. The strong link between the number of blistering sunburns and melanoma suggests that the intensity and duration of sun exposure are more important than cumulative exposure. However, melanoma can occasionally occur in non-sun-exposed areas (e.g. mucosal melanomas), indicating alternate mechanisms of tumor development.

An estimated 8–12% of all cases of cutaneous melanoma occur in those with a familial predisposition. The characteristics of familial melanoma include melanoma in at least two generations, and a family member with multiple primary melanomas or younger age at diagnosis. Affected patients typically will have multiple (>10) dysplastic nevi, although not all melanomas in these patients arise from the pre-existing nevi. Familial melanoma has been variously named familial atypical multiple mole-melanoma (FAMM), dysplastic nevus syndrome, and atypical mole syndrome.

TABLE 13.1. Risk factors for Melanoma.

Fair skin
Red/blonde hair
History of blistering sunburn
Increased number of nevi
Freckles
UV radiation exposure
Family history of melanoma

Implicated genetic mutations include CDKN2A located at 9p21, CDK4 located at 12q14, MC1R located at 16q24, and a mutation of the short arm of chromosome 1 located at 1p22.TP53 and BRAF mutations are reportedly common in melanoma. Thus far, the only commercially available genetic test for melanoma is an assay for mutation of the p16 tumor-suppressor gene (CDKN2A), which accounts for about 40% of heritable melanomas.

Clinical Presentation and Diagnosis

All suspicious cutaneous lesions should be biopsied. The ABCD criteria are a good rule of thumb in identifying which lesions warrant further investigation. These criteria include Asymmetry, Border irregularity, Color variation, and Diameter > 6 mm. Any new or changing lesion, non-healing ulceration, or lesion that appears different from the patient's other nevi also warrants investigation.

Biopsy Techniques

Because biopsy of suspicious lesions should be planned with the goal of definitive diagnosis and future treatment, the biopsy technique should ensure that the sample will be representative of the lesion, and that the deepest portion of the lesion will be evaluable by the pathologist. Excisional biopsies are preferable because the entire lesion can often be removed, allowing the pathologist to examine its full depth. Excisional biopsy should not be undertaken without consideration of the potential for a wide re-excision. Extremity incisions should be longitudinal. Failure to achieve sufficient depth in a biopsy can complicate determination of the overall Breslow thickness of a lesion, making proper staging difficult. Shave biopsies, while common, often fail to adequately sample the deepest portion of the lesion, and therefore, should be avoided except by those who have considerable experience with the shave technique. A punch biopsy or incisional biopsy can be sufficient to establish a melanoma diagnosis for large lesions or lesions in areas where excisional biopsy is undesirable (e.g. face). The specimen from an incisional biopsy should include areas of darkest pigment or the thickest portion.

Preoperative Evaluation

Biopsy evidence of melanoma should be followed by a thorough history and physical examination that includes a full-body skin check to identify any other suspicious lesions and a careful examination of all lymph node basins. All patients with invasive melanoma should undergo chest radiography to rule out pulmonary metastases. Palpable suspicious lymph nodes should be assessed by fine-needle aspiration (FNA). Ultrasound guidance, when available, may aid in sampling the most suspicious area of the lymph node. If the FNA specimen is positive for tumor, a PET/CT with a brain MRI may be indicated to search for metastatic disease elsewhere in the body. Laboratory tests should include a complete blood count and liver function tests including lactate dehydrogenase (LDH); an elevated LDH value may increase suspicion of metastases elsewhere.

Staging

Staging of melanoma is based on the lesion depth, lesion ulceration and the presence and extent of metastatic disease (Table 13.2). Depth of invasion is measured as the Breslow thickness in millimeters from the surface of the lesion. The Clark level of the primary lesion (Fig. 13.2) is most useful to indicate the risk of metastasis from thin lesions; a Clark level of IV or V increases the risk of nodal metastasis. Clark level is more difficult to evaluate than Breslow depth and requires an experienced pathologist. Other stage-related features of the primary lesion include site, mitotic rate per square millimeter, lymphatic or blood vessel invasion, and evidence of regression.

The size (microscopic or macroscopic) of nodal metastases and the number of tumor-involved nodes are important prognostic features. For distant metastases, the location of the metastases impacts survival. Skin, subcutaneous or distant lymph node metastases (M1a) and lung metastases (M1b) carry a substantially better 1-year survival than metastases in other visceral sites (M1c): 59% and 57% vs 41%, respectively.

Management of Primary Melanoma

Wide local excision remains the mainstay of therapy. Failure to obtain adequate margins increases the risk of local recurrence to as high as 40%. The extent of surgical margins has been controversial. Historically, a 5 cm tumor-free margin of tissue around the primary melanoma was considered ideal. Since then multiple clinical trials have demonstrated that a narrower tumor-free margin can result in similar long-term survival. We use radial margins of 0.5 cm for melanoma in situ, 1 cm for thin melanomas (Breslow depth < 1 mm or Clark level < III), 2 cm for intermediate-thickness melanomas (Breslow depth 1–4 mm or Clark level III–IV), and 2–3 cm for thick melanomas (Breslow depth > 4 mm or Clark level V).

TABLE 13.2. American Joint Committee on Cancer Staging of Melanoma and 5-year survival.

Stage	5-Year survival (%)	TNM staging	Criteria
()	>97	Tis	Melanoma in situ
IA	>95	T1aN0M0	≤1 mm without ulceration
IB	89–91	T1bN0M0	≤1 mm with ulceration or Clark level IV or greater
		T2aN0M0	1.01–2 mm without ulceration
IIA	77–79	T2bN0M0	1.01–2 mm with ulceration
		T3aN0M0	2.01–4 mm without ulceration
IIB	63–67	T3bN0M0	2.01–4 mm with ulceration
		T4aN0M0	>4 mm without ulceration
IIC	45	T4bN0M0	>4 mm with ulceration
IIIA	63–69	T1–4aN1aM0	Any thickness, non-ulcerated, 1 lymph node with micrometastases
		T1–4aN2aM0	Any thickness, nonulcerated, 2–3 lymph nodes with micrometastases
IIIB	30–53	T1–4bN1aM0	Any thickness, ulcerated, 1 lymph node with micrometastases
		T1–4bN2aM0	Any thickness, ulcerated, 2–3 lymph nodes with micrometastases
		T1–4aN1bM0	Any thickness, non-ulcerated, 1 lymph node with macrometastases
		T1–4aN2bM0	Any thickness, non-ulcerated, 2–3 lymph nodes with macrometastases
		T1–4a/bN2cM0	Any thickness, any ulceration, in-transit or satellite metastases without lymph node involvement

(continued)

TABLE 13.2. (continued)

Stage	5-Year survival (%)	TNM staging	Criteria
IIIC	24–29	T1–4bN1bM0	Any thickness, ulcerated, 1 lymph node with macrometastases
		T1–4bN2bM0	Any thickness, ulcerated, 2–3 lymph nodes with macrometastases
		T1–4a/bN3M0	Any thickness, any ulceration, ≥4 lymph nodes, matted nodes, or combination of intransit/satellite metastasis and lymph nodes
IV	6–19	T1–4a/bN0–3a-cM1a	Any thickness, any ulceration, any lymph node status, skin/subcutaneous or distant lymph node metastasis
		T1–4a/bN0–3a-cM1b	Any thickness, any ulceration, any lymph node status, lung metastasis
		T1–4a/bN0–3a-cM1c	Any thickness, any ulceration, any lymph node status, other organ metastasis or metastasis with elevated LDH

In cosmetically sensitive areas such as the face, margins may sometimes be narrowed based on the location and stage of the primary melanoma. Punch biopsies along the planned margins can aid in determining the extent of excision (Fig. 13.3). For subungual melanomas, amputation of the distal interphalangeal joint is typically necessary to achieve a reasonable margin; more extensive lesions may require amputation of the entire digit.

Primary closure via simple advancement flaps is usually achievable, but rotation flaps and skin grafts should be used whenever necessary to allow adequate margins for large primary lesions. Either split-thickness or full-thickness skin

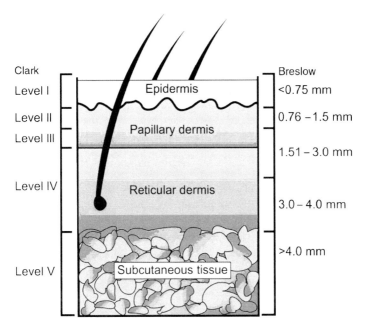

FIGURE 13.2. Correlation between Clark level and Breslow thickness of a primary cutaneous melanoma.

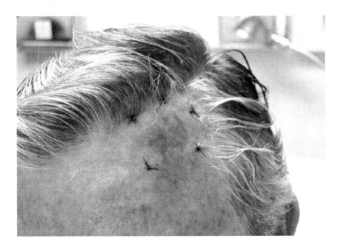

FIGURE 13.3. Serial punch biopsies can be used to evaluate potential margins of excision around a primary cutaneous melanoma.

grafts can provide excellent coverage. We generally reserve full-thickness grafts for scalp and face reconstructions, often harvesting the graft from the posterior neck or anterior chest. Flap reconstruction should be deferred if the surgeon is concerned that the margin may not be negative, because re-excision may jeopardize the entire flap.

Management of Regional Lymph Nodes

The management of regional lymph nodes is primarily surgical in nature. A careful physical exam is key to the diagnosis of regional disease. Ultrasound can be a useful adjunct to clinical exam in detecting metastases. However, in those with a raised suspicion for lymphatic disease, a pathologic examination continues to be the most sensitive method of detecting metastases.

Sentinel Lymph Node Biopsy

The most common site of melanoma metastasis is the regional lymph nodes. Historically, significant controversy surrounded the role of elective lymphadenectomy for the presumed draining lymphatic basin for each melanoma. The potential for lymphedema and other morbidities was balanced against improved staging and locoregional control. The development of intraoperative lymphatic mapping and sentinel lymph node biopsy (SNB) by Morton and colleagues allows minimally invasive surgical staging of clinically localized melanoma. Briefly, SNB is performed by intradermal injection of a radiocolloid and a vital blue dye at the site of the primary tumor. These tracers are carried by the lymphatic system to the draining lymph node basin, where they identify first-order lymph nodes, the so-called sentinel nodes. Although blue staining is still considered the gold standard for identification of a sentinel node (Fig. 13.4), measurement of radioactivity by a hand-held gamma probe can facilitate identification of all sentinel nodes in a drainage basin. Each probe-identified sentinel node should have a radioactivity count of at least 10% of the

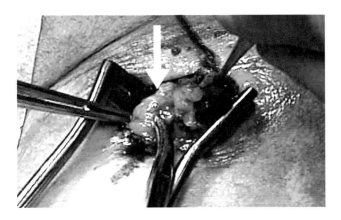

FIGURE 13.4. Blue staining identifies the sentinel node.

most radioactive node.

Sentinel nodes are excised and examined for evidence of metastases. Multiple permanent sections of each node should be stained by hematoxylin and eosin (H&E) and by immuno-histochemistry (IHC) with antibodies for MART-1, S100, or HMB-45. IHC can identify small tumor deposits missed by H&E. Evaluation of frozen sections is discouraged because of potential loss of tissue during processing. If the sentinel node specimen is positive, then complete lymphadenectomy is undertaken; if sentinel nodes are negative for tumor, then no further nodal surgery is necessary.

Prior to SNB, patients should undergo preoperative lymphoscintigraphy to identify the lymphatic drainage basin and the approximate site of sentinel nodes within that basin. Careful examination of the lymphoscintigram can identify aberrant or unusual patterns, such as drainage to popliteal or epitrochlear nodes, or drainage to basins across the midline from the tumor.

SNB should be undertaken in all patients whose primary melanomas are >1 mm and in patients who have thinner melanomas accompanied by risk factors such as a Clark level ≥ IV, ulceration, incomplete biopsy, evidence of regression, high mitotic counts, and young age.

Complete Lymph Node Dissection

There has been little debate about the utility of therapeutic lymphadenectomy in patients with palpable nodes; 5-year survival rate of those with clinically palpable disease is 25–40% depending on the number of nodes involved. For patients with nonpalpable nodes, there has been more controversy; a large phase III randomized multicenter trial is underway to determine whether SNB alone is sufficient in certain patients with evidence of sentinel node metastases. Until the results of that trial are available, complete lymph node dissection is indicated for any basin that contains a tumor-positive sentinel node.

For head and neck lesions, complete nodal dissection generally entails a modified radical neck dissection that can spare the functional structures, although a superficial parotidectomy is often necessary. In axillary dissections, all three levels of nodes including those medial to the pectoralis minor should be resected. In the inguinal region, a superficial lymph node dissection should include the highest femoral node (Cloquet's node) and tissue anterior to the abdominal fascia above the inguinal ligament. If Cloquet's node is positive for tumor, a deep lymph node dissection is undertaken through a second incision or by transecting the inguinal ligament.

The morbidity of complete lymphadenectomy is site-dependent. Wound infections and seromas remain the most common complications. Lymphedema is a vexing problem that is most common in inguinal node dissections; 2–10% of patients experience chronic lymphedema.

Melanoma of Unknown Primary

As many 14% of melanoma patients with nodal metastases are diagnosed without evidence of a primary lesion. A careful search for the primary lesion should include mucosal and ocular examination, as well as a thorough history with regards to prior skin tag excisions or lesions that may have regressed.

Even if a primary lesion cannot be identified, median survival is generally equivalent or superior to that for patients with a similar number of tumor-positive nodal metastases from a known primary site.

Management of Regional In-Transit Disease

When melanoma recurs dermally or subcutaneously between the primary and regional lymphatic basin, it is in-transit metastasis (stage IIIB/IIIC). Because in-transit metastasis is a harbinger of systemic disease within 6–12 months, the overriding goal of therapy is to minimize morbidity. Surgery should be reserved for those with few lesions, and amputation should be considered rarely and as a last resort.

Bacille Calmette-Guérin (BCG) has been reported to control in-transit metastasis in up to 80% of patients when injected intralesionally. Other immunologic adjuncts include injections of human monoclonal antibodies to gangliosides GD2 and GM2 as well as interferon-α. Imiquod, a topical immunomodulator, has also been used with some success. All of these modalities induce a local inflammatory response that may cause the lesion to regress. Larger lesions that shrink but do not disappear should be excised.

Limb perfusion may be an option when extensive in-transit metastases make excision impractical. Since its introduction in the 1950s, this technique has alternately gained and lost favor over the years. The typical method is to isolate a limb by vascular control and infuse hyperthermic melphalan arterially at 42°C while perfusing the affected limb through an oxygenator circuit. Tumor necrosis factor-α (TNF-α) has more recently been combined with melphalan and is approved for such use in Europe. A number of smaller and single-institution studies for patients with very bulky primary and metastatic disease report complete response rates of around 50% with melphalan alone and 75% with melphalan plus TNF-α. The theoretical advantages of limb perfusion are the ability to infuse tumor-toxic doses of chemotherapeutic agents with less-severe systemic side-effects. With careful attention to vascular exclusion, leakage of chemotherapy agents into the systemic circulation is minimal. Limb loss is a rare complication. More recently, percutaneous limb infusion has been used as a simplified method of achieving similar results.

Management of Systemic Disease

Surgical Options

Median survival of patients with metastatic melanoma ranges between 4 and 12 months depending on the M-stage; 5-year overall survival rate is 5.5% at our institution. Because chemotherapy and immunologic therapies provide only limited benefit, metastasectomy should be considered whenever feasible. Metastasectomy should also be considered for symptom palliation in patients with gastrointestinal bleeding/obstruction and CNS mass effect or bleeding.

The most common metastatic sites beyond the regional lymphatics are lung, intestine, liver, and brain. However, because any location in the body can harbor metastatic melanoma, a high index of suspicion should be maintained for any abnormality in a patient with a history of melanoma. Our institutional series has demonstrated 5-year survival rates of 29% in selected patients undergoing complete excision of all metastatic deposits.

Selection of patients should be based on the operation's technical feasibility, the patient's physiologic status, and the tumor's biology. The tumor doubling time is a powerful prognostic factor for the likelihood of durable remission. Tumor doubling time can be calculated from two measurements on radiologic images such as chest x-ray or CT scans (Fig. 13.5). Metastasectomy is unlikely to prolong the survival of patients whose tumors have rapid doubling times(<40 days). Other relative contra-indications include multiple organ sites of metastases, the inability to resect all metastatic tumor, and extreme age or significant co-morbidities. Thorough staging includes a CT of the chest, abdomen, and pelvis, an MRI of

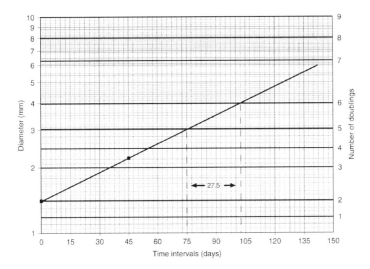

FIGURE 13.5. Tumor doubling time calculation on logarithmic graph paper. The slope of the line is the rate of tumor growth; the doubling time is the horizontal distance (in days) between any two points on the line which correspond to consecutive doublings.

the brain, and a full-body PET scan. These images should be obtained before metastasectomy is considered.

Non-surgical Options

Immunologic Modulation and Targeted Therapies

Immunotherapy has remained the great hope for the future of melanoma therapy, in part because of the occasionally dramatic endogenous immune response to this malignancy. Partial spontaneous regression of the primary melanoma is not uncommon and is accompanied by macrophage and lymphocyte infiltration into the tumor. Although regression is often associated with worse outcomes, the presence of tumor-infiltrating lymphocytes (TILs) is associated with improved survival and decreased risk of sentinel lymph node metastases. In metastatic disease, the reported rate of spontaneous regression is 0.27% of patients; 40% of these regressions are durable. Active specific (vaccine) immunotherapy for melanoma continues to be examined in the adjuvant setting and for systemic disease; however, despite promising results in single-institution phase I and II trials, no vaccine has yet demonstrated improved survival in a randomized phase III trial.

The only FDA-approved immunotherapies for melanoma are interferon-α (IFN-α) and interleukin-2 (IL-2). Adjuvant use of IFN-α after complete excision of disease has yielded mixed results in randomized trials. A pooled analysis of the Eastern Cooperative Oncology Group (ECOG) trials E1684 and E1690 demonstrated a statistically improved relapse-free survival, but not improved overall survival. Meanwhile, the toxicity of IFN-α is high, with the most common side effects being fatigue, flu-like symptoms, and gastrointestinal disturbances. IL-2 when used as a single agent is also significantly toxic in high doses. Reported response rates reach 15%. The 6.6% of patients with complete regression often have a long-term durable response.

Among the targeted therapies under investigation are a monoclonal antibody against CTLA-4 (cytotoxic T lymphocyte-associated antigen 4), a BRAF tyrosine kinase/multikinase inhibitor, and antisense RNA to the proto-oncogene Bcl-2. Patients with stage IV melanoma should be encouraged to enroll in appropriate clinical trials designed to improve therapies for metastatic melanoma.

Chemotherapy

Although dacarbazine (DTIC) remains the only FDA-approved chemotherapeutic agent for metastatic melanoma, its efficacy as a single agent is poor at best; a recent phase III trial demonstrated a 7% response rate and a <1% complete response rate. These rates are not improved by combining

DTIC with nitrosoureas, platinum analogs, or tubular toxins. Temozolomide is a drug that converts to 5-(3-methyltrizen-1-yl) imidazole-4-carboxamide (MTIC), the active metabolite of DTIC. Its primary advantage over DTIC is its oral formulation. Because of its ability to penetrate the CNS, it is also potentially useful for CNS metastases, although the largest trials to date have been for patients without CNS metastases.

Combination Biochemotherapy

The failure of single-agent/multiagent chemotherapy or immunomodulation to elicit long-term responses has led some investigators to combine these strategies into a biochemotherapy regimen. Single-institution trials have demonstrated response rates as high as 60% and complete remission rates of 12–15%, albeit short-term with only 5–10% durable response rates. Randomized cooperative trials of a combination of DTIC and interferon-α showed no additional benefit over DTIC alone. Moreover, the toxicity of biochemotherapy requires inpatient administration and prevents its use for patients with significant physiologic impairment.

Radiation Therapy

The traditional perception of melanoma as a relatively radioresistant tumor has been challenged by reported palliation of symptoms and high (50–70%) response rates with radiotherapy. When anatomic considerations prevent complete excision with adequate margins, as maybe the case for recurrences in head and neck and axillary lymph nodes, radiation can be used as an adjuvant to improve local control and disease-free survival. However, adjuvant radiation is generally unnecessary after adequate complete excision, with the exception of CNS metastases. Stereotactic radiotherapy with the gamma knife has also been used for first-line treatment of CNS metastases and intermediate-stage choroidal melanomas.

Suggested Readings

Atkins MB, Elder DE, Essner R, et al. (2006) Innovations and challenges in melanoma: summary statement from the first Cambridge conference. Clin Cancer Res 12:2291s–2296s

Balch CM, Buzaid AC, Soong SJ (2001) Final version of the American Joint Committee on Cancer staging system for cutaneous melanoma. J Clin Oncol 19: 3635–3648

Morton DL, Ollila DW, Hsueh EC, et al. (1999) Cytoreductive surgery and adjuvant immunotherapy: a new management paradigm for metastatic melanoma. CA Cancer J Clin 49:101–116

Morton DL, Wen DR, Wong JH, et al. (1992) Technical details of intra-operative lymphatic mapping for early stage melanoma. Arch Surg 127:392–329

Morton DL et al. (2008) Multicenter Selective Lymphadenectomy Trial Group: Sentinel node biopsy versus nodal observation for primary melanoma. N Engl J Med (in press)

O'Day S, Boasberg P (2006) Management of metastatic melanoma 2005. Surg Oncol Clin N Am 15:419–437

Rigel DS, Carucci JA (2000) Malignant melanoma: prevention, early detection, and treatment in the 21st century. CA Cancer J Clin 50:215–236

14

Soft Tissue Sarcomas of the Extremities and Chest Wall

Eugene A. Choi and Raphael E. Pollock

Pearls and Pitfalls

- Sarcomas represent a rare heterogeneous group of tumors. Most are derived from embryonic mesoderm; a few arise from ectoderm including: peripheral neuroectodermal tumors (PNET), neurosarcomas, and Ewing's sarcoma.
- The majority (>50%) occur in the extremities; two-thirds of these lesions occur in the lower limb, 19% in the trunk (including 1% chest wall), 15% in the retroperitoneum, and 9% in the head and neck regions.
- Sarcomas are staged according to size, depth (relative to fascial plane), and grade, as well as lymph node status (N) and the presence or absence of metastatic disease.
- Histopathologic grade is the most important prognostic factor for predicting metastasis and tumor-related death. The potential for metastasis is 50–60% in high-grade sarcomas compared to 5–10% in low-grade sarcomas.
- The multimodality approach to therapy of soft tissue sarcoma has reduced the rate of amputations to <10% of patients.
- The cornerstone of treatment of soft tissue sarcomas is a two-centimeter negative margin resection including involved surrounding structures.
- Patients with large (>5 cm) or intermediate-to high-grade soft tissue sarcomas should be considered to receive adjuvant radiotherapy.

K.I. Bland et al. (eds.), *Surgery in Breast Cancer and Melanoma*, DOI 10.1007/978-1-84996-435-7_14, © Springer-Verlag London Limited 2011

- Patients with small (<5 cm) high-grade tumors (stage IIB) do not require adjuvant radiotherapy, unless close, positive, or unknown margins are evident or when re-excision is not possible.
- Patients who present with recurrent disease in the extremity or chest wall and those with positive margins after excision, should undergo re-resection along with radiation therapy.
- While adjuvant doxorubicin-based chemotherapy is associated with a modest increase in overall survival, it should be considered for patients with high-grade and large (>5 cm) tumors in the context of a clinical trial.

Introduction

Soft tissue sarcomas of the extremities and chest wall represent a rare heterogeneous group of tumors. They are derived from embryonic mesoderm, or the soft tissues of the body, including fat, muscle, tendon, synovial tissue, and blood vessels; thus, sarcomas can develop in any site in the body including the gastrointestinal tract. The most common histological subtypes are malignant fibrous histiocytoma (MFH) (28%), followed by liposarcoma (15%), leiomyosarcoma (12%), and synovial sarcoma (10%). The majority (>50%) occur in the extremities; two-thirds of these lesions occur in the lower limb, 19% in the trunk (chest, abdomen, back, shoulders), 15% in the retroperitoneum, and 9% in the head and neck regions.

Incidence and Etiology

It is estimated that in 2007 approximately 11,590 new sarcoma cases were diagnosed in the United States, and 4,890 will die from this disease. According to the National Institute of Health and Surveillance Epidemiology and End Results (SEER) database, from 2000 to 2003, the median age at presentation was 56 and the median age at death was

65. The incidence of soft tissue sarcoma is similar between men (3.6 per 100,000) and women (2.6 per 100,000) among all ethnicities.

Most sarcomas have no clearly defined etiology; however, sarcomas have been associated with certain chemical exposure such as phenoxyacetic acids, which are found in herbicides, and chlorophenols, which are found in pesticides, and in small amounts in chlorinated water. Other chemicals that have been associated with the development of sarcoma include dioxin, vinyl chloride, and Thorotrast. The relationship between radiation exposure and lymphedema followed by the development of soft tissue sarcoma has been well described. While the risk of sarcoma depends on the radiation dose, patients typically present with latent sarcomas within 10 years. Breast cancer patients who have undergone mastectomy and axillary dissections and who received postoperative radiation therapy may develop persistent lymphedema, predisposing them to the development of angiosarcomas (Stewart-Treves syndrome).

Genetics

There are also genetic variables which predispose individuals for the development of soft tissue sarcomas. *In vitro* studies have demonstrated that mesenchymal stem cells can acquire mutations in oncogenes *N-myc*, c-erbB2 and *ras*, as well as in tumor suppressor genes including p53 and RB-1, which can result in cell proliferation and survival despite accumulation of cellular genetic mutations. In addition to mutations in tumor suppressor genes, cytogenic abnormalities have been described. For example, in Ewing's sarcoma, there is translocation t(11;22)(q24;q11.2–12) and in synovial sarcoma, translocation t(X;18)(p11.2;q11.2). Genetic syndromes such as neurofibromatosis (NF) and familial adenomatous polyposis (FAP) are associated with the development of sarcomas. Patients with FAP develop intra-abdominal desmoid tumors that are often located in the small bowel mesentery.

Clinical Presentation

Sarcomas are often asymptomatic and come to clinical attention after an antecedent episode of trauma of the involved area. In one-third of the cases, patients present with pain. Sarcomas are often mistaken for intramuscular hematomas, lipomas, and sebaceous cysts, which results in a delay in the correct diagnosis. Symptoms typically develop when the sarcomas become large (>10 cm). In the extremities, lesions may invade the deep investing fascia and neurovascular structures, leading to swelling and pain; with retroperitoneal sarcomas, involvement of the gastrointestinal tract can cause obstructive symptoms or displacement of the diaphragm and produce symptoms of gastroesophageal reflux (GERD). Soft tissue sarcomas of the chest wall typically present with pain or as an asymptomatic mass that may appear in the breast. Given the rarity of the tumors, a high index of suspicion is required to make the correct diagnosis.

Evaluation of the Symptomatic Patient

The key to the correct diagnosis begins with a comprehensive history and physical examination. The physician must assess the mobility of the mass in relation to the surrounding tissues; in addition, attention must be paid to the size, depth, and consistency of the mass. Draining lymph node basins and the overlying skin should be examined for metastatic disease. In extremity sarcomas, motor and sensory function of the affected extremity and signs of swelling should be documented. Previous exposure to radiation or certain chemicals should be included in the history. Needless to say, one should inquire about personal and family history of malignancy or genetic disorders.

Staging

The staging of sarcomas has undergone some changes in the past several years. Sarcomas are staged according to size, depth (relative to investing fascia), grade, lymph node status

(N), and the presence or absence of metastatic disease (see Table 14.1). Histopathologic grade depends on the following: cellularity, differentiation, necrosis, pleomorphism, and mitosis. The current American Joint Committee on Cancer (AJCC) staging system for soft tissue sarcomas is designed

TABLE 14.1. American Joint Commission on Cancer staging of soft tissue sarcoma (From American Joint Committee on Cancer, 2002. With permission).

Primary tumor (T)

TX	Primary tumor cannot be assessed
T0	No evidence of primary tumor
T1	Tumor 5 cm or less in greatest dimension
	T1a Tumor above superficial fascia
	T1b Tumor invading or deep to superficial fascia
T2	Tumor more than 5 cm in greatest dimension
	T2a Tumor above superficial fascia
	T2b Tumor invading or deep to superficial fascia

Regional lymph nodes (N)

NX	Regional lymph nodes cannot be assessed
N0	No regional lymph node metastasis
N1	Regional lymph node metastasis

Distant metastasis (M)

MX	Distant metastasis cannot be assessed
M0	No distant metastasis
M1	Distant metastasis

Histopathologic grade (G)

GX	Grade cannot be assessed
G1	Well differentiated
G2	Moderately differentiated
G3	Poorly differentiated

(continued)

TABLE 14.1. (continued)

Histopathologic grade (G)		
Histopathologic grade (G)		
G4	Undifferentiated	
Stage grouping		
A	G1–2, T1a-1b, N0, M0	(Low grade, small, superficial, deep)
B	G1–2, T2a, N0, M0	(Low grade, large, superficial)
Stage II		
A	G1–2, T2b, N0, M0	(Low grade, large, deep)
B	G3–4, T1a-1b, N0, M0	(High grade, small, superficial, deep)
C	G3–4, T2a, N0, M0	(High grade, large, superficial, deep)
Stage III	G3–4, T2b, N0, M0	(High grade, large, deep)
	Any G, any T, N1, M0	(Any metastasis)
Stage IV	Any G, any T, N0, M1	

for lesions of the extremity, but can be applied to lesions of the trunk, head and neck, and retroperitoneum. However, the staging system does not apply to visceral sarcomas, desmoids, and dermatofibrosarcoma protuberans.

Several investigators have identified that histopathologic grade is the most important prognostic factor for predicting metastasis and tumor-related death. The risk of distant metastasis is 50–60% in high-grade sarcomas compared to 5–10% in low-grade sarcomas. However, the staging system limits itself by stratifying patients according to their risk of distant metastases, but not necessarily for risk of local recurrence.

Imaging

The preferred imaging for sarcomas of the extremity is magnetic resonance imaging (MRI). MRI delineates the tissue planes between masses, neurovascular structures, and normal tissue planes. However, a recent study by the Radiology Diagnostic Oncology Group (RDOG) comparing MRI and computed tomography (CT) scan in 367 patients showed no difference between the two imaging modalities in terms of predicting soft tissue mass involvement with bone, joint, or neurovascular structures. Some practitioners often use both imaging modalities to collect complementary information about tumors. CT scans are more helpful for chest and intra-abdominal (visceral and retroperitoneal) sarcomas, and current CT scans can provide three-dimensional reconstructions. Furthermore, CT scan is an equivalent alternative for patients who cannot undergo MRI, specifically patients with pacemakers and metal prostheses. There has been growing interest in the use of fluorodeoxyglucose positron emission tomography (FDG-PET) as another imaging modality for soft tissue sarcomas of the extremities. This technique may be helpful in defining high- and intermediate-grade sarcomas.

In addition to diagnostic imaging performed for the primary tumors, complete staging work-up should include a chest radiograph (see Fig. 14.1). Patients with low-grade or high-grade sarcomas less than 5 cm require a chest radiograph; any questionable lesion(s) or suspicion of metastatic disease on chest radiograph requires a contrast-enhanced spiral CT.

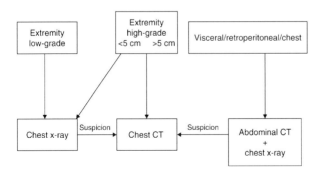

FIGURE 14.1. Algorithm demonstrating staging work-up for sarcoma (Reprinted from Brennan and Lewis, 2002. With permission).

Patients with high-grade (II or III) extremity sarcomas greater than 5 cm require a chest CT as the first imaging test. Extremity, truncal, and head and neck sarcomas often metastasize to the lungs, while intra-abdominal sarcomas metastasize to the liver. Attention to nodal involvement on cross-sectional imaging is important, as this may be seen in less than 5% of patients, particularly in patients with histological subtypes such as epithelioid sarcoma, angiosarcoma, clear cell sarcoma, synovial sarcoma, and rhabdomyosarcoma.

Biopsy

The histological types and subtypes of soft tissue sarcomas determine both prognosis and treatment design. Therefore, obtaining tumor tissue diagnosis is generally required in the preoperative setting. There are various techniques for biopsy including fine-needle aspiration (FNA), core needle biopsy, and excisional and incisional biopsy. For superficial palpable lesions, core needle biopsy can be performed safely in most circumstances, and for deeper lesions, ultrasound and CT scan can help facilitate core needle biopsy. FNA is an equally effective method, but is not routinely performed because it requires the expertise of cytopathologists who regularly evaluate sarcoma tissue. FNA is often performed to diagnose recurrent disease.

Patients with superficial small (<3 cm) lesions may undergo excisional biopsy in place of a needle biopsy. If percutaneous-based procedures fail to provide a diagnosis, an open biopsy is an alternative method of diagnosis. Ideally, an incisional biopsy should be performed by the same operative surgeon who would perform the definitive resection. The incision should be oriented parallel to the long axis of the extremity to facilitate subsequent wide local excision of the tumor, biopsy site, and incision en bloc. In general, when planning an open biopsy located on the extremity, trunk, or head and neck, the incision should be carefully planned, in consideration of the subsequent local management of the tumor.

Treatment

Treatment is determined by the histopathology and stage of the sarcoma, as well as patient preferences and expectations (see Fig. 14.2). Thus, treatment of soft tissue sarcoma utilizing a multimodality approach is best provided at specialized cancer centers. In the simplest case, a patient presenting with a low-grade sarcoma of the extremity which is located away from vital neurovascular structures can undergo negative margin surgical resection. However, a patient with a high-grade sarcoma located deep within the medial thigh can be presented with different treatment options, including (1) surgical resection for pathologic staging and postoperative radiotherapy, (2) preoperative external beam radiotherapy

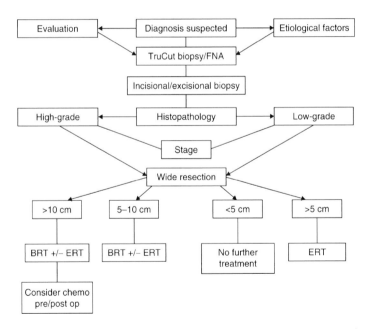

FIGURE 14.2. Algorithm for the evaluation and treatment of extremity soft tissue sarcoma. (Reprinted from Brennan et al., 2001. With permission).

with subsequent surgery, (3) protocol-based chemoradiation treatment followed by consolidation surgery, or (4) induction of intermediate-to high-dose anthracycline-based chemotherapy with preoperative radiation and subsequent surgical resection.

Surgery

The primary treatment modality for localized soft tissue sarcomas is negative margin resection. In the past, patients with sarcomas of the extremity have undergone amputation. However, the surgical approach has transformed into one of limb-sparing operations. In one of the landmark prospective trials, the National Cancer Institute (NCI) randomized 91 patients with high-grade extremity sarcomas into amputation versus wide local excision and adjuvant radiation. Although patients who underwent limb-sparing treatment developed higher rates of local recurrences, the overall 5-year survival rates between limb-sparing treatments (83%) versus amputation (88%) was not statistically different. This development of a multimodality approach to soft tissue sarcoma has reduced the number of amputations to <10% of patients.

Surgical Principle

The goal of resection is to resect the mass and any involved structures with a two-centimeter rim of normal tissue. A margin of less than 2 cm may be considered appropriate if the sarcoma is in close proximity to neurovascular structures or juxtaposed near bone. Sarcomas should never be enucleated because of a high risk of local recurrent disease. Any previous incisions from biopsy or previous surgery should be resected, as there is a chance of local recurrence from tumor seeding. Further, the treatment modalities for patients with chest wall soft tissue sarcomas are similar to that for extremity sarcomas.

For chest wall sarcomas, surgical treatment may involve rib and sternal resections, and adjacent thoracic structures. A multi-specialty approach allows for reconstruction with rotational flaps supported by synthetic materials where necessary (see Fig. 14.3).

Surgical technique is critical, as studies have demonstrated margin-negative (R0) resection as a prognostic factor for local recurrence rate and disease-specific survival. Sarcomas of the extremity and superficial trunk/chest wall which are low-grade and < 5 cm in size are often cured with wide resection alone. To achieve a R0 resection, surgery may require the expertise of several disciplines including vascular, reconstructive, head

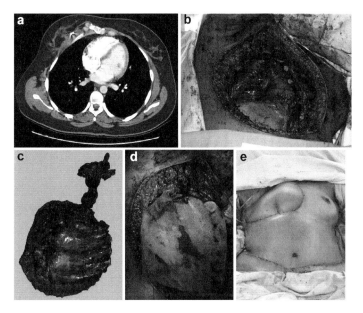

FIGURE 14.3. Resection of recurrent chest wall soft tissue sarcoma. **a**. Preoperative cross-sectional imaging of the right chest wall demonstrating recurrent disease and postoperative changes. **b**. Operative field after en-bloc resection of the right chest wall mass, and second, third, fourth, and fifth. **c**. Resection specimen. **d**. Chest wall defect with reconstruction with Marlex mesh. **e**. Flap closure of chest wall defect.

and neck surgery, and neurosurgery. For patients who present with recurrent disease in the extremity or chest wall or positive margins after excision, re-resection and radiation therapy is recommended.

Radiation Therapy

To improve local control after resection, radiation therapy is delivered to patients with (>5 cm) high-grade sarcomas of all types. Several prospective, randomized trials have demonstrated the efficacy of adjuvant radiation. The NCI evaluated the role of radiation therapy with wide local excision. Eligible patients with high-grade sarcomas were randomized to undergo wide local excision and adjuvant chemotherapy versus surgery and radiation therapy with chemotherapy. The investigators demonstrated a significant decrease in local recurrences in patients who received radiation therapy. However, this approach did not impact overall survival. Similar results were seen in patients with low-grade sarcomas who received surgery alone versus surgery combined with adjuvant radiation treatment. Patients with small (<5 cm) high-grade tumors (stage IIB) do not require adjuvant radiotherapy unless for close, positive, or unknown margins or when re-excision is not possible.

Brachytherapy

Despite the proven effectiveness of adjuvant external beam radiation therapy (EBRT), there remain questions about the most effective method of radiation delivery, the optimal dose, and the timing (preoperative or postoperatively). An alternative to adjuvant EBRT is adjuvant brachytherapy (BT), which has several advantages. It can be completed in 4–6 days compared to 4–6 weeks, can be given directly to the tumor bed which limits radiation scatter to vital structures (joints), can improve functional outcome, and in one study, lowers hospital charges.

Pisters et al. evaluated the effectiveness of adjuvant brachytherapy in a single-institution, prospective, randomized trial. Eligible patients (n = 164) with primary or recurrent extremity sarcoma were randomized to receive adjuvant brachytherapy or no adjuvant therapy after limb-sparing procedures. Patients were given 42–45 Gy over 4–6 days with iridium 192. There was an improvement in local control in the brachytherapy arm versus surgery alone, and 13 and 25 local recurrences, respectively. In this trial, brachytherapy had an effect on local control in patients with high-grade tumors only. Adjuvant radiotherapy did not demonstrate any difference in development of distant metastases or in overall survival for both low-and high-grade sarcomas.

Brachytherapy can also be applied in previously irradiated fields to facilitate limb-sparing treatment for recurrent disease. Several groups have combined EBRT with brachytherapy and demonstrated an improvement in local control in patients with stage III disease. However, patients with large (> 5 cm) low-grade sarcomas should be treated with adjuvant EBRT.

Preoperative External Beam Radiotherapy

The interest in preoperative radiation therapy for extremity soft tissue sarcomas has evolved for several reasons: (1) to avoid tumor hypoxia (undisrupted blood supply), (2) to reduce the radiation fields with possible better functional outcomes, and (3) to sterilize the primary tumor, improve resectability, and reduce the likelihood of iatrogenic tumor seeding. A few studies have demonstrated that preoperative radiation therapy may be beneficial in decreasing local recurrence in patients with large tumors (>15 cm) or with gross disease on presentation. However, the single randomized prospective trial comparing pre-and postoperative radiation in patients with extremity sarcomas showed no difference in local recurrence, metastatic disease, or overall survival. A higher rate of postoperative wound complications was noted in patients who received preoperative radiation therapy. However, this complication may be avoided with the utility of flap reconstruction.

Adjuvant Chemotherapy

The introduction of radiation therapy has increased limb-sparing procedures and decreased local recurrence. However, the natural history of patients with extremity soft tissue sarcomas is to develop metastatic disease. As in other solid tumors, adjuvant chemotherapy has been used to prevent the development of metastatic disease and related mortality. Several systemic agents have been effective against sarcomas including doxorubicin, cyclophosphamide, ifosfamide, cisplatin, methotrexate, dacarbazine, and etoposide. The three most widely used agents are doxorubicin, ifosfamide, and dacarbazine, with response rates, as determined by radiographic tumor shrinkage, between 17% and 25%.

The use of single agent adjuvant systemic chemotherapy, specifically with doxorubicin, has not been effective in preventing local recurrence and improving disease-free and overall survival. To increase the response rate of sarcomas, various combination chemotherapy regimens have been studied. Most of the regimens tested included an alkylating agent, an anthracycline (doxorubicin), and/or dacarbazine. However, studies comparing combination chemotherapy regimens to observation alone have also failed to consistently provide an improvement in overall survival. Unlike single agent chemotherapeutic protocols, combination therapy trials have shown trends toward improvement in local recurrence and disease-specific survival.

Studies that evaluated single therapeutic agents did not show any benefit due to the small study numbers. In addition, the staging method and histological grade among the individual studies were inconsistent to reach definitive conclusions. A recent meta-analysis of 14 studies including 1,568 patients with localized, resectable soft tissue sarcoma reported by the Sarcoma Meta-analysis Collaboration showed improvement in disease-free survival and local disease-free survival at 10 years in the doxorubicin-based adjuvant chemotherapy arm with a median follow-up of 9.4 years. However, there was no difference in overall survival. In a subset of the 866 patients with extremity sarcoma, chemotherapy was associated with a modest increase in overall survival.

Adjuvant chemotherapy should not be routinely used. With the introduction of more effective chemotherapy agents such as ifosfamide and gemcitabine, and the development of supportive hematopoietic growth factors, adjuvant chemotherapy may provide benefit, but should be performed in the context of a clinical trial. Patients with large tumors (>5 cm) of intermediate-or high-grade should be considered for adjuvant chemotherapy.

Neoadjuvant Chemotherapy/Isolated Limb Perfusion

There has also been interest in preoperative chemotherapy and chemoradiation, which may provide a clinical response to achieve negative margin surgical resection. The advantage of such an approach is that non-responders to chemotherapy are spared further postoperative treatment. Several studies have proven that preoperative chemotherapy and chemoradiation followed by wide local resection for extremity soft sarcomas increase overall, local, and distant disease-specific survival compared to historical controls.

For unresectable disease, a limb-sparing alternative treatment modality is isolated limb perfusion. This procedure involves cannulation of the arterial and venous blood supply to the extremity connected to a pump oxygenator for regional administration of high-dose chemotherapy, specifically melphalan and tumor necrosis factor(TNF) under hyperthermic conditions. However, the response rates have been variable from 18% to 80%. This variation in response to isolated limb perfusion is believed to be due to the heterogeneity of the patient demographics, tumor location, and characteristics.

Follow-up

In the aftermath of curative resection, patients with extremity and chest soft tissue sarcomas will typically develop local recurrence or metastatic disease during the first 2 years.

Therefore, patients with high-grade sarcomas should be followed every 3–4 months during the first 2 years and every 4–6 months thereafter with regular imaging studies. We typically ultrasound the resection site, as well as obtain a MRI (for extremity sarcomas), or CT scan (for trunk/chest wall and retroperitoneal sarcomas) and a chest radiograph at the time of follow-up for surveillance. Patients with small <5 cm or low-grade sarcomas can be followed every 6 months for the first 5 years and annually thereafter. Annual chest radiograph should be considered for small or low-grade lesions.

Outcomes

In one of the largest series, patients with extremity soft tissue sarcomas treated with wide local resection had a 5-year overall survival of 76% with a local recurrence rate of 17%. Two hundred twenty-four patients (22%) developed distant disease. Two-thirds of the tumors were high-grade and located in the proximal lower extremity underneath the investing fascia. In spite of the location and histopathology of the tumors, a great majority (>80%) of patients underwent limb-sparing surgery without adjuvant chemotherapy or radiation. Despite advances in strategies implementing radiation and chemotherapy, the overall and disease-specific survival rates have remained unchanged in the past 10 years.

Review of the published studies of patients with primary soft tissue sarcomas of the chest wall has demonstrated 5-year overall survival rates have ranged from 65% to 87.3%, with local recurrence rates at 5 years from 10% to 27%, and rates of metastases from18% to 35%. There was a slight predominance of low-grade (53%) tumors compared to high-grade tumors (47%), and higher survival rates were associated with low-grade sarcomas.

The differences in overall survival, local recurrence rates, and rates of metastases may reflect the differing proportion of low-and high-grade sarcomas, as well as differences in pre-and postoperative treatment patients received relative to surgical resection in individual studies. Overall, patients who presented with chest wall or extremity sarcomas and underwent wide local excision had similar survival rates.

Conclusion

Sarcomas represent a rare heterogeneous group of tumors. While the vast majority of sarcomas occur in the extremities, sarcoma can be found throughout the body. Current AJCC staging encompasses criteria based on size, grade, depth, lymph node status, and distant disease. Grade represents the most important predictor of survival and disease recurrence. Surgical resection is the only known curative treatment; however, radiation and chemotherapy may have benefit only in select cases. A multimodality approach is recommended for lesions >5 cm, lesions in proximity to vital structures, or lesions that require complex reconstruction for optimal functional and cosmetic outcomes.

Selected Readings

American Joint Committee on Cancer (2002) AJCC Cancer Staging Manual, 6th edn. Springer-Verlag, New York, www.springeronline.com

Andrews SF, Anderson PR, et al. (2004) Soft tissue sarcomas treated with postoperative external beam radiotherapy with and without low-dose-rate brachytherapy. Int J Radiat Oncol Biol Phys 59:475–480

Athanassiadi K, Kalavrouziotis G, et al. (2001) Primary chest wall tumors: early and long-term results of surgical treatment. Eur J Cardiothorac Surg 19:589–593

Brady LW, Kramer S, et al. (2001) Radiation oncology: contributions of the United States in the last years of the 20th century. Radiology 219:1–5

Brennan MF, Alektiar KM, Maki RG (2001) Sarcomas of soft tissue and bone. In: Devita VT, Hellman S, Rosenberg SA (eds) Cancer: principles and practice of oncology, 6th edn. Lippincott, Williams & Wilkins, Philadelphia

Brennan MF, Lewis JJ (2002) Diagnosis and management of soft tissue sarcoma. Martin Dunitz, London

Gordon MS, Hajdu SI, et al. (1991) Soft tissue sarcomas of the chest wall. Results of surgical resection. J Thorac Cardiovasc Surg 101:843–854

Grobmyer SR, Daly JM, et al. (2000) Role of surgery in the management of postmastectomy extremity angiosarcoma (Stewart-Treves syndrome). J Surg Oncol 73:182–188

Heslin MJ, Lewis JJ, et al. (1997) Core needle biopsy for diagnosis of extremity soft tissue sarcoma. Ann Surg Oncol 4:425–431

Janjan NA, Yasko AW, et al. (1994) Comparison of charges related to radiotherapy for soft-tissue sarcomas treated by preoperative external-beam irradiation versus interstitial implantation. Ann Surg Oncol 1:415–422

Meric F, Milas M, et al. (2000) Impact of neoadjuvant chemotherapy on postoperative morbidity in soft tissue sarcomas. J Clin Oncol 18:3378–3383

Panicek DM, Gatsonis C, et al. (1997) CT and MR imaging in the local staging of primary malignant musculoskeletal neoplasms: Report of the Radiology Diagnostic Oncology Group. Radiology 202:237–246

Pisters PW, Harrison LB, et al. (1996) Long-term results of a prospective randomized trial of adjuvant brachytherapy in soft tissue sarcoma. J Clin Oncol 14:859–868

Pisters PW, Leung DH, et al. (1996) Analysis of prognostic factors in 1,041 patients with localized soft tissue sarcomas of the extremities. J Clin Oncol 14:1679–1689

Rosenberg SA, Tepper J, et al. (1982) The treatment of soft-tissue sarcomas of the extremities: prospective randomized evaluations of (1) limb-sparing surgery plus radiation therapy compared with amputation and (2) the role of adjuvant chemotherapy. Ann Surg 196:305–315

Stewart FW, Treves N (1981) Classics in oncology: lymphangiosarcoma in postmastectomy lymphedema: a report of six cases in elephantiasis chirurgica. CA Cancer J Clin 31:284–299

Yang JC, Chang AE, et al. (1998) Randomized prospective study of the benefit of adjuvant radiation therapy in the treatment of soft tissue sarcomas of the extremity. J Clin Oncol 16:197–203

Index